COMPASSION FATIGUE AND BURNOUT IN NURSING

Vidette Todaro-Franceschi, RN, PhD, FT, has been a nurse for 30 years and has worked in a variety of acute and long-term care settings in medicine, surgery, and critical care as staff nurse, administrator, clinical specialist, educator, and consultant. She is an associate tenured professor and coordinator of the Clinical Nurse Leader Graduate Program at Hunter-Bellevue School of Nursing, Hunter College, and Doctoral Nursing Faculty at the Graduate Center, both of the City University of New York. A nurse scholar and educator in the areas of end-of-life/palliative care, bioethics, and leadership, Dr. Todaro-Franceschi is the author of the book *The Enigma of Energy: Where Science and Religion Converge* along with many articles and several chapters. She has performed seminal research on ideas of energy, synchronicity, bereavement healing, end-of-life care, and professional quality of life. A passionate speaker, she has presented nationally and internationally.

Dr. Todaro-Franceschi is an End-of-Life Nursing Education Consortium (ELNEC) trainer and a Fellow in Thanatology (ADEC). She is on the academic advisory board for *Annual Editions: Death, Dying and Bereavement,* and is a peer reviewer for a number of professional journals including the *Journal of Hospice and Palliative Nursing, MedSurg, Nursing Science Quarterly,* the *Journal of Holistic Nursing,* and *Alternative Therapies in Health and Medicine.*

COMPASSION FATIGUE AND BURNOUT IN NURSING
Enhancing Professional Quality of Life

Vidette Todaro-Franceschi, RN, PhD, FT

SPRINGER PUBLISHING COMPANY
NEW YORK

Springer Publishing Company, LLC
11 West 42nd Street
New York, NY 10036
www.springerpub.com

Acquisitions Editor: Allan Graubard
Composition: Techset Composition Ltd., Salisbury, UK

ISBN: 978-0-8261-0977-4
E-book ISBN: 978-0-8261-0978-1

12 13 14 15/5 4 3 2 1

The author and the publisher of this Work have made every effort to use sources believed to be reliable to provide information that is accurate and compatible with the standards generally accepted at the time of publication. Because medical science is continually advancing, our knowledge base continues to expand. Therefore, as new information becomes available, changes in procedures become necessary. We recommend that the reader always consult current research, specific institutional policies, and current drug references before performing any clinical procedure or administering any drug. The author and publisher shall not be liable for any special, consequential, or exemplary damages resulting, in whole or in part, from the readers' use of, or reliance on, the information contained in this book. The publisher has no responsibility for the persistence or accuracy of URLs for external or third-party Internet Web sites referred to in this publication and does not guarantee that any content on such Web sites is, or will remain, accurate or appropriate.

Library of Congress Cataloging-in-Publication Data

Todaro-Franceschi, Vidette.
  Compassion fatigue and burnout in nursing : enhancing professional quality of life / Vidette Todaro-Franceschi.
    p. ; cm.
  Includes bibliographical references and index.
  ISBN 978-0-8261-0977-4 -- ISBN 978-0-8261-0978-1 (e-book)
  I. Title.
  [DNLM: 1.   Nurses--psychology. 2.   Burnout, Professional--psychology. 3.   Empathy.
  4.   Philosophy, Nursing. 5.   Quality of Life. WY 87]
  610.73--dc23

                                                    2012023136

Special discounts on bulk quantities of our books are available to corporations, professional associations, pharmaceutical companies, health care organizations, and other qualifying groups.

If you are interested in a custom book, including chapters from more than one of our titles, we can provide that service as well.

For details, please contact:
Special Sales Department, Springer Publishing Company, LLC
11 West 42nd Street, 15th Floor, New York, NY 10036-8002s
Phone: 877-687-7476 or 212-431-4370; Fax: 212-941-7842
Email: sales@springerpub.com

Printed in the United States of America by Bang Printing

Dedicated to my colleagues—
nurses everywhere—and especially my students . . . .
May you always work heartfully, *assured that those whose lives*
you touch will be forever changed.

CONTENTS

Part 5   Beating the Odds

FOREWORD

In her classic work, *Ordered to Care*, historian Susan Reverby (1987a) wrote about the roots of nursing as a predominantly women's profession. Women were expected to take care of infirmed close and distant relatives. When caregiving moved outside of the home, it was women who were expected to provide it. Indeed, it was one of the few occupations open to women. Caregiving was viewed as "women's work"—a view that we continue to challenge today—and, as such, was not valued by society. Reverby (1987b) argues that nurses have been, and continue to be, ordered to care in a society that refuses to value caring. Her work helped many in nursing to understand the complexity of the profession and nurses' own views of self-worth and their conduct. How can we feel good about the work we do if it is not valued by society?

When society devalues what we do, it is hard to clutch the thread that holds together the tapestry of caring. Nursing is extremely demanding and challenging work. We are witnesses to tremendous trauma, both physical and psychological. The work takes its toll when we, our colleagues, and the health systems in which we work fail to understand that caring for the caregivers is essential if we are to provide high-quality, humanistic care.

We sometimes do our work in uncaring environments. Our health care system is notorious for failing to deliver the right care in the right way at the right time. Hospitals are often more concerned about nurses administering medications than making sure that patients and their family caregivers have the information and support they need to be able to take care of themselves in the immediate post-discharge period. Physicians continue to give "orders," as if they had the certitude of the Ten Commandments, even though our duty is to the patient first. Nurses who challenge the status quo or the "orders" of physicians quickly learn that they can be disciplined and even lose their jobs and livelihood. They leave work knowing that they have been unable to support patients in ways their patients needed. Whether it is from unsafe systems of care, insufficient staffing to provide the care patients and families need, or being constrained from advocating for patients as our conscience dictates and our heart demands, too many nurses lose their compassion and move from embracing their work as heroic and profound to viewing it as a job they just need to get through each day. Far too many remain in practice but have lost the compassion that is central to excellent nursing care.

Increasingly, nurses are rejecting society's devaluation of nursing care and are embracing the profound nature of their work. Nursing focuses on the human condition, not merely disease. We are with patients during some of their most vulnerable, intimate, terrible, and joyous times of their lives. We help patients to live healthier lives, to recover from debilitating illnesses, and to make the transition from life to death. We pride ourselves in caring for individuals, families, and communities. And, let us be clear: "Caring" is not simply being nice; it requires exquisite knowledge, skill, compassion, and insight.

Now is the time for nurses to be bold in acting on a vision for a caring health care system. Nursing and health care are entering a new era that holds the promise to transform this system in ways that will benefit nurses, other health care providers, and the people they serve. This movement is accelerating because of two recent developments:

- The Institute of Medicine's (2010) report on *The Future of Nursing: Leading Change, Advancing Health* provides our nation with a synthesis of the evidence documenting our worth—whether as staff nurses who are the last barrier from errors reaching the patient, school nurses who detect potentially deadly contagions before they can spread throughout a community, home care nurses who improve the quality of lives of patients and reduce health care costs by preventing hospital readmissions, advanced practice nurses who help patients to live healthier lives, or public health nurses who ensure that families are able to live in safe environments. The report is framed as what must be done to ensure that our nation is able to provide access to quality, equitable, affordable health care by strengthening the largest of the health care professions—nursing. The Robert Wood Johnson Foundation, which funded the report, is working with AARP to move forward the report's recommendations at the national and state levels. The stakeholders in this work include business groups, patient advocacy organizations, insurers, health care organizations, and nursing organizations, among others. This is a game changer for nursing and society.

- The Affordable Care Act is the first large-scale attempt to transform our inefficient, fee-for-service health care system that fails to deliver on quality, health outcomes, and cost. It seeks to shift the system from a focus on expensive high-tech, acute care to one that prioritizes health promotion, prevention, and chronic care management. While the health reform law is imperfect, it provides multiple avenues for turning around a huge system that our nation can no longer afford. Nurses are central to its success.

We need help in rising to meet the challenges these two milestones present. One important resource is this book, *Compassion Fatigue and Burnout in Nursing*, by Vidette Todaro-Franceschi, RN, PhD, FT. It provides nurses with a guide to understanding how to never let go of the centrality of compassion and caring to nursing and their work by taking care of themselves, valuing their work, refusing to let others diminish their worth, and creating the conditions in which caring can thrive. The book is a must-read for all nurses—not just those who are burned out. As Dr. Todaro-Franceschi notes, we must take care of ourselves if we are to take good care of people. Doing so requires that we lead the creation of caring communities of work. It cannot be acceptable for a hospital, or a nursing home, or school of nursing to be a caustic well of heartlessness. Places that claim to provide health "care" must walk their talk by creating healing environments for those who are ordered to care. But these environments are *us—you and me*. We have the opportunity—and, I would argue, the responsibility—to ensure that we and our workplaces embody the ethos of caring that is central to health and healing. This interesting and readable book provides nurses with the knowledge and tools to seize this opportunity.

I do not want to live in a society that does not value caring. As the profession that has its roots in caregiving, we can no longer accept anything less than compassion nor be silent about unsafe, uncaring health care organizations. Now is the time for nurses to take care of themselves and to lead in transforming health care and society into communities of caring. If we do not, who will?

Diana J. Mason, RN, PhD, FAAN
Rudin Professor of Nursing
Hunter-Bellevue School of Nursing
Hunter College, City University of New York

REFERENCES

Institute of Medicine. (2010). *The future of nursing: Leading change, advancing health*. Washington, DC: National Academies Press.

Reverby, S. (1987a). *Ordered to care: The dilemma of American nursing*. New York: Cambridge University Press.

Reverby, S. (1987b). A caring dilemma: Womanhood and nursing in historical perspective. *Nursing Research, 36*(1), 5–11.

FOREWORD

Nursing—an evolving and maturing profession—is struggling to find its identity, voice, and place, in an increasingly technologically driven and ethically challenging health care environment. We all share a desire to effect positive change, to have our voices heard, and to feel included and significant. Long recognized as a profession grounded in presence, the therapeutic use of self, caring, and compassion, nurses are especially at risk for moral distress, compassion fatigue, and burnout when consistently unable to provide the type of humanistic care that patients and families need. This has become all too common. Yet, centers of excellence do exist where an environment has been created that encourages reflective practice and open and honest communication without fear of retribution.

How do we prepare nurses to enter the present health care environment and support them? Traditionally, time-constrained nurse educators have focused on "fitness to practice" and competencies while self-awareness and reflective practice have received much less attention. Both skill sets are essential for a nurse to feel professionally realized, to fully engage as a member of the health care team, and to advocate for the patient.

With this as a background, Dr. Vidette Todaro-Franceschi, a seasoned clinician and nurse educator, gives a passionate explication of nurses' professional quality of life. Described by her as the Good, the Bad, and the Ugly, she takes a personal historical perspective using her own decades of experiences as a bedside nurse caring for the dying, and a nurse educator of both graduate and undergraduate students. Dr. Todaro-Franceschi uses anecdotes—both her own and those of her students—to illustrate factors that influence a nurse's professional quality of life and contribute to compassion fatigue and burnout. Through the use of these stories, nurses are helped to recognize the pressures and forces that influence their practice, and the feelings of powerlessness and erosion of integrity that may arise from the inability to control conditions of their practice and employment. Dr. Todaro-Franceschi explores how to constructively approach these forces and to turn them into something that is positive rather than leading to anger, frustration, and burnout. Education in clinical ethics, communication, mediation and advocacy, as well as assertiveness training and working as a team member, are all components.

This is a strongly written book that will resonate with many nurses—not only bearing witness to their distress and giving voice to their experiences but also providing constructive steps to move forward.

Nessa Coyle, RN, ACHPN, PhD, FAAN
Consultant, Palliative and End-of-Life Care and Clinical Ethics

PREFACE

I woke up one day, after years in practice, and realized I did not look forward to my time at work anymore. It was a subtle change that took place over time and then WHAM! It hit me. I hated going to work and in one of my disillusioned moments during my nursing career, I decided to apply for a job outside of nursing. It was at a time when we really did not need the money; financially we were doing fine. I had been working as a staff nurse in critical care for several years and I was not happy. Do not get me wrong; I love nursing. I was just tired of seeing people so sick, often dying. Tired of working every other weekend, every other holiday, knowing full well that we would be short-staffed and I would not be able to take a break or, more importantly, provide the quality care that I wanted to give to my patients. Tired of getting talked down to by the occasional pompous physician, and well, I was just plain *tired*. So, I applied for a job at Macy's.

I went in to their personnel department on my day off, while the kids were in school, filled out the paperwork, and took a short test. I did not mention it to my husband or friends; I knew they would not understand. A week later they called me to schedule an interview at which time they offered me a supervisory position. They said I was "over qualified" to be a salesperson. Hmm, I thought. I could easily switch careers and get a great shopping discount to boot. I seriously thought about it, for all of one day.

When I sat down to dinner that night and told my husband about my interview and the Macy's offer, you could have put quarters in his eye sockets. He said, "Are you crazy? Are you kidding? Why would you leave nursing to work in Macy's?" Of course, he was right. How could I consider throwing away my nursing career? We discussed at length my options. Shortly thereafter, I applied and then enrolled in graduate school, and cut back from full- to part-time work for a while. It was not a permanent fix, I knew. Eventually I changed positions altogether. In fact, during my almost 30-year career, I have changed positions frequently;

just about every time I felt myself slipping, that is to say, becoming more automated and less humane. I was fortunate that I was not afraid of change and have never felt locked into any one job.

Years later, as a nurse educator, I realized that there was a repeating theme in the often-voiced reasons why nurses came back to school. Many seemed to be suffering from varying degrees of compassion fatigue, although they were unaware of it. So I started to incorporate content related to professional quality of life in courses I was teaching and, unsurprisingly, every time the topic came up I received a dramatic response.

There has been very little focus on this important issue in nursing education or practice settings. Yet, it seems that compassion fatigue in health care is universal and crosses all cultural boundaries, and nurses, as frontline carers, are the most vulnerable.

A while back I presented a paper titled *Preventing Compassion Fatigue: Reaffirming Purpose in Nursing* at the European Federation of Critical Care Nurses Congress/Aniarti Conference in Florence, Italy (Todaro-Franceschi, 2008). I did not expect the volume of people that came to hear my presentation. Over 600 nurses attended—there was standing room only. And at least a third of the people in attendance were in tears at the end of my presentation. Later that day when I spoke again, this time on communicating with the dying and their loved ones, over 1000 nurses attended.

For the rest of my time in Florence I was regularly approached in the street, restaurants, and stores by conference attendees who wanted to thank me for "clearing their heads," "helping them to find the purpose they felt they had lost," and in general assisting them to remember why they chose a nursing career in the first place. A few noted that they had never realized what was happening to them and one said, "now I know what is wrong with some of the people where I work." Comically, whenever we were alone, my husband, who accompanied me on the trip to Italy, kept shaking his head and saying, "I didn't know I was married to a rock star!"

That humbling experience provided a big AHA! moment for me. In nursing we are *individually* and *collectively* craving to retain our sense of purpose. Nurses need to be aware of this phenomenon—compassion fatigue and the related syndrome of burnout—that is infecting the nursing workforce like a plague. What's more, we need to know what can be done to heal from it and, when possible, how to side-step it. But the answer to our individual and collective woes in nursing does not lie solely in an exploration of compassion fatigue and poor professional quality of life. To fix the problem, we need to look at the bigger picture. We need to explore the reason why we each chose to embark on the path we now find ourselves: in lifelong service as nurses.

Thus, this book is really about compassion and contentment. It is about what led us into a caregiving profession—into nursing. It is about reconnecting with the meaning and purpose of our life's work. It is hoped that having read this book, you will return to work, renewed in spirit and resolved to help others, so that together we can reaffirm purpose in nursing and health care.

Author's Note: The terms "burnt out" and "burned out" are used interchangeably throughout the book.

ACKNOWLEDGMENTS

T he seed for this book was planted many years ago but really came to fruition while I was on sabbatical and at Hastings Center as a visiting scholar roaming through its wonderful library, participating in lunch discussions, sharing ideas, and renewing myself on its beautiful grounds in Garrison, New York. Thank you, Dan Callahan for creating this wondrous space where dialogue and reflection on some of the most important issues related to living–dying are valued and encouraged. Appreciation also goes to Thomas H. Murray and all the staff at the Center for making me feel welcome.

Gracious thanks goes to Kenneth Doka, Professor of Gerontology at the Graduate School of The College of New Rochelle, who introduced me to Sheri W. Sussman, Executive Editor at Springer Publishing, who in turn enthusiastically encouraged me to submit a book proposal. Thanks also goes to Allan Graubard, Executive Acquisitions Editor, who guided me from start to completion, Christina Ferraro, assistant editor, who nudged me as necessary, Michael O'Connor, Senior Production Editor, who answered my many queries, and Nick Barber, who did the typesetting. I would also like to thank Joseph DePinho the graphic artist, who, when I asked that there be a butterfly on the cover, provided a beautiful one with the most perfect colors—a real synchronicity!—along with the rest of the staff at Springer who worked on this project.

Much appreciation also goes to valued colleagues Margaret Lunney and Nessa Coyle, who each took time from their busy schedules to read early drafts of Chapters 1 and 2, and provided me with useful feedback. Gratitude also goes to my wonderful student and research assistant Maddie Hubbell who put together a great resource list, much of it is included at the end of the book. I had to eventually tell her to halt—she was so dedicated to the project.

Occasionally I hear from students who tell me how well I taught them—they should know that they taught me well too. Teaching and learning is always reciprocal. My appreciation to the many students and nurses who have shared their stories over the years is humbly expressed through this publication and is a heartfelt wish for their happiness.

Lastly, much love and gratitude go to my family; Ernest and Charlotte Todaro, who taught me the value of education; Ginn, Laura, and Tara, who each in their own ways supported me; and, Mikey, Dette, and Nicky, for always bringing me joy and respite when needed. And as always, Michael, no words can express my appreciation as I once more stole precious time from you and our family to lock myself in a room working. Thank you too, for being my sounding board, and for inspiring and sharing ideas. This would not have happened without you.

COMPASSION FATIGUE AND BURNOUT IN NURSING

Part 1

PROFESSIONAL QUALITY OF LIFE

Professionally speaking, are you alive or just lingering? Are the people who work with you or for you thriving or barely surviving? If the quality of your professional life is questionable, prolonging it may be a grave disservice. There are worse things than death for a person or a professional. If you have to make a choice, go for quality.
—MELODIE CHENEVERT

Chapter 1

INTRODUCTION: THE GOOD, THE BAD, AND THE UGLY

Our prime purpose in this life is to help others.
And if you can't help them, at least don't hurt them.
—DALAI LAMA

KEY TOPICS

Introduction to positive and negative aspects of professional quality of life:
- Compassion contentment
- Compassion fatigue
- Burnout

Nurses know all about "quality of life." It is the main focus of our profession—we provide care to enhance the quality of our patients' lives. However, many nurses may not know that their *own* quality of life is at stake, depending upon how they go about their work each day. Indeed, a lot of nurses, although familiar with the terms *compassion fatigue* and *burnout*, cannot identify how it manifests or whether they or their co-workers are experiencing it.

Countless individuals have emphasized the potential detriment to self that can arise from the unique work of health care professionals. However, psychologist and scholar Beth Stamm (2002, 2010) has paid equal attention to the positive aspects of professional quality of life. In looking at the negative consequences of providing care, she came to realize that not everyone who witnesses suffering when caring for others actually develops compassion fatigue; many people still manage to go about their work in a joyful manner. Thus, she expounds upon three components of professional quality of life: *compassion satisfaction, compassion fatigue,* and *burnout* (Stamm, 2002, 2009, 2010).

The positive aspect of professional quality of life, what Stamm (2002, 2010) refers to as compassion satisfaction, is derived from doing caring work and readily manifests itself as happiness, or at the very least, contentment, in the workplace. It is the pleasure that one gets from helping others (Stamm, 2002). I rather like the term *compassion contentment*, for it seems to better allude to a sense of pleasure, something greater than "satisfaction," which to me could be merely passable.

When we can appreciate our work as meaningful, we feel content. Stamm's (2002) approach to professional quality of life can be useful for those who are interested in fostering healthy work environments, particularly in light of all the work being done with appreciative inquiry as a means of enabling and enhancing constructive change in organizations. With appreciative inquiry one focuses on the positive aspects of things rather than the negative, in order to come to understand what can be done to replicate the good and, in so doing, diminish the bad.

Compassion fatigue and burnout are the two most frequently talked about aspects of professional quality of life. Nurse Carla Joinson (1992) first used the term *compassion fatigue* in nursing when writing about the negative feelings that nurses sometimes experience while caring for people who are suffering. She wisely noted that "compassion fatigue is almost impossible to recognize without a heightened awareness of it" (p. 116), and while 20 years later we know this to be the case, we still do not insist that our nursing workforce and leadership be well versed in this area. In fact, there is a great deal of conflicting information in the accumulating literature on the subjects of compassion fatigue and burnout; sometimes the terms are used interchangeably, and in the early literature, compassion fatigue was simply a form of burnout specific to carers (nurses, physicians, therapists, etc.). In much of the later writings on the subject, however, the two syndromes have been described as distinct entities, and in this book, I, too, differentiate between them.

Although each may contribute to the other, compassion fatigue and burnout are different in how they come about and manifest in each of us. I will make a disclaimer here that I am not attempting to reconcile any discrepancies in the literature; instead of getting caught up on terminology, I want to get right to what I perceive to be the essence or *heart* of the matter.

The nurse's overall professional quality of life is important for both the carers *and* the recipients of care. They are one, so the heart of the matter is *heart*. Heart is a synonym for many pertinent words; if you look at a thesaurus, you will find that it can also mean compassion, empathy, kindness, sensitivity, and spirit, among other love-conjuring terms.

I think of people who love caring for others and are content doing their work as *heartful*, and I cannot help relating it to the spiritual aspects of human nature. For me, spiritual denotes a sense of belonging to everything else in the universe and to each other. It encompasses the scientific but makes subjective aspects (for instance, how we feel and what we think) just as essential, and sometimes even more so, than the objective (what we can see and measure) aspects of existence. People who are *heartful* tend to be more aware of their connection to everything else.

Compassion fatigue is relational in nature, meaning it arises through one's relationships with others. Typically, compassion fatigue manifests suddenly while caring for those who are suffering from any kind of physical or mental anguish or trauma. The suffering rubs off on the carers and can be, as Joinson noted, "emotionally devastating" (1992, p. 116). A social worker who has talked and written about the subject, Karl La Rowe, refers to compassion fatigue as having *a heavy heart* (Perry, 2008, p. 87), a description I find most applicable and one that I use throughout the following pages.

Whereas compassion fatigue is related to our connection to others and our ability to bear witness to the suffering of others, burnout arises out of a more generalized dissatisfaction with one's work life, and it is usually the result of a multitude of things. Of course, one's relationship with others can be a big factor, but workload, environment, salary, benefits, organizational culture—many things can set the stage for burnout. Burnout develops gradually over time with prolonged emotional and physical exhaustion, and it ultimately results in widespread apathy, a disinterest in work and relationships (Maslach, 1982).

People who are burned out and work in health care are frequently seen as *dis*passionate because their apathy appears to indicate a lack of caring. In other words, they appear *heartless* (or *empty hearted*) and usually feel quite hopeless (dis*heart*ened!) to make things better in their work lives. The feelings of discontent that may arise from one's work and which lead to the development of burnout can, and frequently do, spill over into our personal lives. If we are not mindful, it can even snuff the enjoyment out of our daily living (and can also remove the joy from our loved ones' lives in the process!). So when I refer to the good, the bad, and the ugly of professional quality of life, I am referring to *compassion contentment*—heartful (the good); *compassion fatigue*—heavy hearted (the bad); and *burnout*—seemingly heartless or empty hearted (the ugly).

HEARTFUL, HEAVY HEARTED, AND HEARTLESS

We definitely cannot afford to be ostensibly heartless and yet I repeatedly hear from students that what they are seeing out there in their clinical practicums and work environments is a workforce that seems predominantly empty hearted. The display of dispassionate care can be extremely disturbing, especially to undergraduate students, and it can be challenging trying to put it all in context. At different times in our lives, each of us may be heartful, heart heavy, or seemingly empty hearted or heartless. The point is, in nursing we really need to be heartful, at least most of the time—it is a matter of health and healing for us as well as those we care for.

I often share the story of John Doe, a homeless young man who had been found unresponsive on a street corner, and who quickly went from being simply unresponsive without a known diagnosis into full-blown multisystem failure (Todaro-Franceschi, 2008a, 2011a). We had no health history, no name, and consequently no family or friends to call. I was assigned to care for John during the first night tour that he was on our unit. He was a one-to-one patient, his care acuity being high enough to warrant one nurse to work with him for a full shift.

John had tubes for everything: a central line, an arterial line, a Foley catheter, a nasogastric tube for feeding, and he was intubated and on a respirator. He was dirty, really dirty. There was caked muck under his nails and toenails and in his hair. There was dirt between his fingers and toes and even in his eyebrows. That first night I spent a significant amount of time bathing him, trying to remove all the grime; I only partially succeeded.

I wondered about him; he was a fairly nice-looking young man, with dark blonde hair and gray-blue eyes. How did he come to be homeless? Did he have family members somewhere who wanted to know where he was and who would be there right now holding his hand if they did know? What caused him to be so ill? How might we help him? How might I help him? I quickly realized that aside from maintaining the status quo in terms of trying to keep him stabilized, the only thing I could do was acknowledge his humanness by talking to him as I cared for him and trying to ensure that he was as comfortable as possible.

John was assigned to me the following two nights and they were difficult, to say the least. He had not regained consciousness. He was on multiple intravenous (IV) medications, which I was constantly titrating up and down to maintain homeostasis; but that was not the hardest part of caring for John. The most difficult thing was to see unrealized potential, to watch a human being who was clearly dying without loved ones, without us knowing who he was and had been. I continued to talk to him as I cared for him, and each night I took over where the day tour nurse had left off, as we each slowly and painstakingly removed what appeared to be years of dirt and grime from his body.

This was a week when I was scheduled to work four nights in a row and I had difficulty sleeping when I went home. As I drove back to work, I dreaded the thought of caring for John another shift, and when I reported to the unit for my fourth consecutive tour, the charge nurse started to assign me to work with him again. I began to cry and told her I simply could not spend another night in the room with him; it was just too painful. I was fortunate in that our charge nurse was an understanding leader and she quickly made out a new assignment for me.

That night, John coded and I ended up in his room for much of the shift, helping a coworker who had been assigned to care for him. I felt so terrible, for both the patient and my coworker. John was pronounced dead after several tortuous hours of trying to keep him alive. When we did postmortem care we removed the little remaining dirt; he was finally clean. In a way, his cleanliness had a sad element attached to it too, for by having removed the last vestiges of grime, in a way it erased what was known about who he was and how he had lived.

My coworker and I consoled each other; we had done everything humanly possible to save our John Doe. As I drove home that morning, I was comforted with knowing I had talked to him and cleaned him as best I could. Perhaps, by my having done so, John had, on some level, been aware that he was cared for by another human being. After all, it is said that hearing is the last sense to go. On autopsy they found that he had contracted leptospirosis, a serious disease carried by various animals and spread through contaminated water, food, or soil.

Twenty years later, I can still see John ever so clearly in my mind. I recognized years ago that, at that time, I was suffering from compassion fatigue. It is possible that I was experiencing a bit of death overload too, having been working in critical care and bearing witness to many deaths by that time. I also realize, in retrospect, that John was, in part, the reason for my shift in focus; he was a turning point for me. I went from critical care nursing to a focus on care of the dying. Most notably, I have come to appreciate that cases like John and so many other individuals that I have worked with over the years, by their sustaining memory, continually help to reaffirm a sense of purpose, a sense that there is always a reason why I do the things I do as a carer. I know that if I keep that sense of purpose first and foremost in my mind, it guides me to always do whatever I do with compassion and, I might add, passion.

The story of John is an example of the good, the bad, and what could have turned out to be ugly. My being able to bear witness to his suffering—cleaning him, touching him, speaking with him—these were actions that get at compassion contentment. My dreading the thought of working with him one more night was indicative of my ability to suffer with, to internalize the anguish of the John Does in this world who die young and alone with strangers; I quickly manifested compassion fatigue. Had my charge nurse been less of a leader, she might not have changed my assignment, creating a bigger wound that could have festered over time, contributing to eventual burnout. The wound would have been bigger, because, without her sincere acknowledgment of my hurting—my humanity—I would have certainly felt worse than I did.

Compassion fatigue can be healed and many times even averted if we are mindfully aware of how we are acting in the workplace (Todaro-Franceschi, 2008a). If we can take note of the things that scare us and the ways we are acting, for instance, my dreading going to work to care for John or being overly upset by the suffering of particular patients and/or their loved ones, we can mindfully care for ourselves to ensure our own well-being.

GOING TO THE PLACES THAT SCARE US

We all have sustaining memories that, on occasion, pop into our awareness. It is important to reflect upon them and consider what our past experiences have contributed to who we are today, even if it means reliving difficult times in our lives. Pema Chodron (2001), an American Buddhist nun, explains that we need to *choose* to go to the places that scare us. By learning to be fearless, we can grow and develop more fully our compassionate nature. If we, in nursing, are unwilling to go, or can no longer go, to the places that scare us (or if we always circumvent around those places, for example, we do not like to care for people who are dying or perhaps we choose not to make eye contact with them or their loved ones), then we have work to do in order to heal from and/or prevent compassion fatigue.

That fourth night going into work, I was distressed at the thought that I would have to care for John yet another shift. It was a place that scared me. As a critical care nurse, having had many experiences with patients who were close to death, I was still terribly uncomfortable with dying and death at times. Watching him die was very hard for me.

Most of us in nursing have gotten the impression somewhere along our professional life journey that it is not right to be distressed or to refuse an assignment, when really we should be okay with our discomfort, because after all, we are humans, not robots—we think, we feel, we hurt, we laugh, and we love. We should be more than okay with speaking up and saying, I just *cannot* do this now. Everyone, leaders and educators, as well as staff—all of us—need to keep prominently in mind that we *are* human beings as we go about the many times overwhelmingly difficult job of nursing; we *all* have our limits. Knowing this, then, can help us remain true to ourselves and our intrinsic caring nature.

Recognizing our limitations and our own distress is very important, so even while we may occasionally say, "I cannot do this now," by acknowledging that where we are right now in this moment *is* a place that scares us, we are, in reality, facing it and embracing it as part of our own humanness. That is *always* a good thing, not a bad thing.

TURNING POINTS

Various experiences lead to turning points in our lives. Turning points are occasionally referred to as critical incidents, and these incidents can be positive or negative. Sometimes we are aware of what has led up to a change in our way of thinking and/or being in the world, but more often than not, the transformation is subtle and we do not take notice. Over time, we subsume our experiences into the core of our being and sometimes we forget who we used to be. It is in looking back that we come to know what has contributed to who we have become. Thus, the goal here is for some of the stories I share to jar *your* memories.

Keep in mind that at the time when many of our most memorable experiences occur, we do not know how important the events will be in the shaping of our careers and lives. For me, it was only through intentional effort to try to make sense of things, usually at times when I felt a bit lost, that I recognized some of my important turning points. That really is the way it happens for many of us, most of the time. Looking back helps us to look forward. Hopefully, as you recall some of your own stories, you will reflect upon how your experiences have changed the way you go about being in the world.

WORKING AGAINST THE ODDS

Nurses who bear witness to human suffering on a regular basis are especially at risk of compassion fatigue; however, there are many things that contribute to the development of diminished professional quality of life. Work conditions—the physical environment as well as organizational culture—can enhance or hinder contentment on the job, and nurses who work in certain areas may be more likely to develop compassion fatigue and/or burnout over time. My own observations and studies have led me to believe that how nurses are educated also plays a significant part in their ability (or inability) to be *heartful* while working.

In an especially telling exploration of what nursing is and the difficulties inherent in the profession of nursing, writer Suzanne Gordon (2005) portrayed us as working *against the odds*. In a lot of ways, we are working against the odds. Chaotic changes in health care systems, attributed in part to the increasing complexity of health care, along with economic constraints, have contributed to the sense that everyone involved in care delivery is working against the odds, and nurses as frontline carers are even more so than any other health care professional. Some of these things are not of our choosing or making, but some of the reasons why the odds seem to be against us definitely are of our making, and I think the way we have been, and continue to be, educated is a big part of the problem. We, in nursing, have to some extent stacked the deck against ourselves.

I want to be clear. I am not pointing an accusatory finger at any one group—no one group owns the current state of affairs in nursing; not staff, educators, or leaders. We are a *collective* body, and we are faced with a crisis in our profession, unlike any other in the history of nursing. We are not dealing with just a shortage of nurses, which is going to worsen as our aging workforce retires. We have issues with recruitment, retention, productivity, unhealthy work environments (which includes a whole other cadre of problems such as incivility and bullying, lack of resources, heavy workload, etc.)—all of these and more are contributing to a crisis that is manifesting in instances of individual and collective compassion fatigue, moral distress, and burnout, but in this era of unprecedented challenges for us in nursing, there is also a collective opportunity.

On the following pages, I hope to illuminate how we can reshuffle that deck individually and collectively and bring some of the missing joy back into nursing. I would like to begin here by pointing to what might make one more than capable of working against the odds—whatever those odds might be. To work against the odds takes passion (or if you prefer, enthusiasm), along with resiliency and maybe more than a little sense of one's own importance. We *have* to believe in ourselves and in what we are about. I do not believe that all, or even most, nurses are educated to believe in ourselves and the power we have collectively as a profession.

No matter what leads to compassion fatigue and burnout, it is clear that some kind of purposeful action is necessary in order to heal from these syndromes, and with adequate knowledge of contributing factors, one may be able to evade the occurrence or at least minimize the effects of compassion fatigue and/or burnout. Thus, the first step is to be able to recognize and acknowledge that there is a problem brewing.

Nurses most likely to quickly relate to the topics explored herein will be those with firsthand experience working with the very ill and dying individuals and their loved ones. Staff nurses and advanced practice nurses who work in emergency rooms, intensive care units, and those who work on medical/surgical, oncology, and palliative care units will easily relate to these topics; however, I believe that most nurses, at some point or another during the course of their career, will experience a degree of compassion fatigue and/or burnout, whether it is due to their frequent exposure to suffering, or to the chaos of their workplace environment, or even more likely, a combination of the two. Consequently, every nurse should have a knowledge of the factors that play a part in how both syndromes can develop and what steps can be taken to facilitate compassion contentment, thereby enhancing professional quality of life and minimizing the potential purportedly negative consequences of our work.

Nurses who work in leadership positions will also benefit from reading this book. I recently had a discussion with a new clinical nurse leader student who works in nursing administration; she asked me, "During this program, will I learn how to motivate my staff?" The answer to that is complex, because in many places, there is collective compassion fatigue and even perhaps collective burnout. I discuss this in further detail later; suffice to say here that leaders cannot hope to motivate staff who have disconnected with the purpose of their work, and in essence, that is what eventually happens to many nurses who suffer from compassion fatigue for any length of time. Accordingly, those who would lead others in health care today need to know how to identify and address the serious workforce woes that impact professional quality of life in order to preserve the integrity and quality of health care, as well as the integrity and quality of life for their staff. It is all one.

Throughout this book, I expound upon each of the three aspects of professional quality of life, and in various instances, I use storytelling; some of the stories are mine and span across my years of nursing practice. Some are narratives that have been imparted by students and friends. Still others are anecdotes about experiences I had as a recipient of care or while witnessing a loved one who was receiving care. All are shared as part of a whole, to get at what it means to be a nurse and to do the actions of nursing.

In the next chapter, I discuss the integral relationship between the cared for and the carers, with an emphasis on an ethic of care which I perceive to be inherent in our discipline. In Part 2, I discuss the positive aspects of our professional quality of life, focusing on compassion contentment and its relationship to our ethical foundation—the values and excellences identified and solidified in our code of ethics. I also introduce a healing model specifically designed to address the enhancement of professional quality of life. Part 3 covers the bad—compassion fatigue; and the ugly—burnout; again, I make no attempt to conciliate what is out there in the literature. Rather, I draw from the literature and my own experiences and observations to put forward ideas related to each of the three components of professional quality of life.

In Part 4, I discuss how facing death can negatively affect us and, conversely, how it can positively transform the way we go about being in the world and how we go about caring for the dying and their loved ones. I include a discussion on collective trauma and death overload, from both natural and man-made disasters, along with post-traumatic stress. In Part 5, the discussion is expanded to include the collective healing of our profession and how, through knowing participation, we can work toward transforming the workplace and enhancing our professional quality of life.

KEY POINTS

- The quality of our professional life is important for us—nurse carers—and equally important for those entrusted to our care.
- Our work contributes to how we go about being in the world, personally and professionally.
- When we are content with our work, it is good and we feel heartful.

- When we internalize suffering, it is bad; we become compassion fatigued and heart heavy.
- When we are discontent and become disconnected from our work, distancing ourselves from others, it is ugly; we are suffering from burnout and are seemingly empty hearted or heartless.
- How we go about our work is important and can provide clues as to what we need to do for ourselves and for others to transform health and healing for all.

Chapter 2

TRANSFORMING BOTH HEALTH AND CARE

It is a beautiful and mysterious power that one human being can have on another through the mere act of caring ... A great truth, the act of caring is the first step in the power to heal.
—PHILLIP MOFFITT

KEY TOPICS

- What is a nurse?
- Ideas of energy, health, and healing
- Unity and purposeful change
- Subtle influences and butterfly power
- Caring in nursing

V ery often we talk about cure of illness, prevention, and promotion of health as the main aspects of health care, but in actuality, it is all about transforming the quality of living and dying. Nurses are instrumental in this transformation. The following story, shared by a student in focused group discussions on end-of-life care, depicts the wholeness of our caring work:

I lost my mom during the summer of 1991, right before my 21st birthday. Her death was a shock to my family and me. She had a severe vomiting episode and fell unconscious after having lunch. For six days she was in a vegetative state, hooked up to a ventilator from a ruptured cerebral aneurysm. She had hemorrhaged badly and the physicians couldn't do anything to help her. My dad had to make the most difficult decision by signing the "Do Not Resuscitate" (DNR) papers. My mom was only 59.

I will never forget Nurse Katie. She made sure my dad had the coveted reclining chair floating on the hospital floor, which was safely tucked away in my mom's room with a "do not remove from this room" sign on it. Nurse Katie made sure my eight sisters and I were allowed to see my mom at the same time during visiting hours, despite the hospital rules. Nurse Katie was 8 months pregnant, wore her sandy, blond hair in a ponytail, and made sure my mom was comfortable. The pain and sorrow I experienced losing my mom was worse than any physical pain I had ever endured. I miss my mom so much and wish she was around to give me a hug. Despite the emptiness I feel not having my mom here, I am grateful my dad had the courage to sign those DNR papers. My mom would've hated spending her remaining days in the hospital, hooked up to a machine while her loved ones suffered, keeping vigil at her bedside.

We brought Nurse Katie a bagful of candy and other treats to show her how much we valued the care she gave to my mom and all of us during our 6 days at the hospital. She cried and hugged us all when my mom's heart stopped beating. Nurse Katie was a gem, and it's nice and reassuring to know that there are other gems just like her out there.

NURSES: PRIMARY TRANSFORMERS IN HEALTH CARE

A question many individuals might ask at this juncture in our professional history, "What is a nurse?" is difficult to answer. Multiple entry levels into practice—the diploma and associate, baccalaureate, master's, and doctorate degrees—combined with so many different titles, can leave even the most well learned on the subject of nursing unable to easily articulate who we are and what it is we do.

In the early days of professional nursing role development, the idea of being "called to care" was readily discernible. Today, for some people, coming into nursing may not be so much a "call to care" as it is about other things, such as job security, a good salary, flexible working hours, multiple opportunities, and so forth. Yet, those of us in nursing and people in the public sector will easily recognize that this student's sustaining memory of Nurse Katie epitomizes what it means to be a nurse.

Nurses assist with healing and are the primary transformers in health care. We are agents of change for individual, group, and community health and healing. Health and healing, in this instance, include all aspects of the life process from birth to death, neither living nor dying being more important than the other, for both are integral with our human becoming.

How do we, in nursing, transform health and assist with healing? While working in critical care, I came to wonder about what it was we were doing, and to me, it appeared related to the idea of energy. *Energy* is one of those terms that we use all the time, but rarely do we ever stop to reflect on its meaning. It has been identified as a foundational concept for all sciences, and as nursing is considered to be a science, it seemed important to be able to understand and explain what it is we mean when we use the word in our work (Todaro-Franceschi, 1998, 1999).

In the intensive care unit (ICU), we were often doing things that to me did not make much sense. For example, nurses would obtain daily weights, no matter how critically ill our patients were. This meant using a Hoyer lift to do bed scale weights. What a frightening experience for those patients who were alert enough to be aware of what was going on, being lifted up on a machine over the bed! What a scary experience for the nurses, too, when the patients were already so unstable!

During my time working in this one ICU, several patients coded during bed scale weighing, and one of them actually died. Consequently, many of us refused to do daily weights on those we believed were unstable, and this resulted in ongoing unpleasant discourse with some of the physicians who wanted those weights everyday no matter what. Thankfully, today, most places have weight scale devices that are built into the beds. However, I would bet that if you reflect on your practice, you could identify similar kinds of practice issues that remain unaddressed and may be contributing to your discontent at work.

The insistence on daily weights and other ongoing events in the ICU setting had me pondering the goals of care, which at the time, seemed to me should encompass conserving energy rather than depleting it. Notably, these kinds of experiences frequently set the backdrop for nurses working in our unit to suffer from what is commonly referred to as moral distress. We had frequent spurts of sick calls, but we all knew that, most of the time, the person calling out sick was really taking a much needed "mental health day."

After taking my own share of mental health days while working on this particular unit, something I had never felt inclined to do before and for which I was feeling extremely guilty, I changed my workplace and eventually went back to graduate school, where I set out to explore ideas of energy. My journey led me through the literature from antiquity up into current-day writings in philosophy, chemistry, physics, cosmology, medicine, psychology, and, of course, nursing (Todaro-Franceschi, 1998, 1999, 2001, 2008b). The takeaway from that exploration is very relevant to the topics in this book, for what emerged was an ethic of care grounded in philosophy but also ubiquitous in the various scientific disciplines.

The Enigma of Energy: A Brief Synopsis

There are two ideas of energy in the literature: a traditional view of energy as part of causal processes, and a more progressive or modern view, where energy is a phenomenon—a thing (Todaro-Franceschi, 1998, 1999). Various disciplines use the term in both ways, but everyone today pretty much agrees that energy is *the* phenomenon that manifests itself into everything we can and cannot see. As Einstein (1954) pointed out in his special theory of relativity, matter and energy are interchangeable. That is to say, for example, that you and I are both manifestations of energy, as is the space between us—with all that is in it—whether we can see whatever is in it or not. It is all essentially *one* thing. He also emphasized that we, the observers of everything around us, are participants in everything around us and, therefore, to a certain degree, we create our reality.

The idea that everything is energy is quite profound when one thinks about it, for it means that there is absolutely no real separation between anything. It implies, too, that "I" or "me" is an utter illusion; one could say there is only "us" or "we." Yet, words cannot quite capture and elucidate the meaning of this enigmatic phenomenon, energy.

It—energy—never stands still. It is always changing forms. Some are natural, like when a caterpillar becomes a butterfly or a fertilized egg becomes a baby, and others are human-instigated, like taking gasoline and using it in fuel lines to transform energy into the motion of a vehicle. Accordingly, one can see that energy transformation occurs *purposefully* and not haphazardly. The changing nature of things is really organized, even when it appears chaotic, and occasionally, if we are lucky, we gleam from what appears to be unpredictable and meaningless behavior, a movement toward something greater than ourselves, an underlying pattern of wholeness—oneness. When one senses this pattern in the whole, it can be a spiritual awakening of sorts for many individuals. I know that I cannot look at anything today without a sense of wonder.

After years of study, I ended up ultimately noting that while the phenomenon of energy will never be fully explained, its mysterious nature nevertheless infers that there is an underlying reason for it all. For how else can you explain something that is every single moment changing purposefully?

HEALTH AND HEALING

Given a pristine appreciation of what I perceived to be the unity and purposeful nature of the universe, I set about exploring health and healing with my new set of glasses. It was no surprise to me that ideas of oneness and purposeful action were there in various writings in medicine and nursing. Hippocrates and Nightingale both wrote about a healing force of nature that seems to cure from within; they were astutely aware of the purposive character of health and healing.

Nightingale (1859/1946) noted, "It is a curious thing to observe how almost all patients lie with their faces turned to the light, exactly as plants always make their way towards the light ..." (p. 49). When discussing healing, she reflected, "It is often thought that medicine is the curative process. It is no such thing; medicine is the surgery of functions, as surgery proper is that of limbs and organs. Neither can do anything but remove obstructions; neither can cure; nature alone cures" (p. 74). She also claimed that it is the nurse's responsibility to "put the patient in the best condition for nature to act upon him" (p. 75).

Health and healing are purposeful manifestations of the one. Health does not mean the absence of disease: One can heal as he or she is dying; one can live until he or she dies, with a good quality of life and in peace. In that sense, one can die healthy. Today, in many sectors of health care, we emphasize healthy aging, as if everyone will live forever; yet, as human beings are living longer and dying slower, there is no doubt that we need to be concerned with "healthy dying" as well as healthy aging. Basically, we must be concerned with healthy *living-dying*, or, if you prefer, the *quality* of living and dying.

Nurses, physicians, and other health care professionals, as well as loved ones, participate in the actualizing of human potential for the individual who is seeking to heal, as they are a part of the whole—the one (Todaro-Franceschi, 1998, 1999). It is in and through all of our purposeful actions that healing arises. That there is unity and purposeful action in all things little and large throughout the universe is the foundation of my ethic of care, for, if it is all essentially one, whatever I do or you do is not just reflected in the whole; *it is the whole.*

In nursing, educators and leaders, of necessity, focus on and emphasize quality and safety issues related to the provision of care. Yes, we all need to be concerned with that; however, one can teach, talk about, and continuously act to try to ensure quality and safety, but if the nursing workforce is compassion fatigued and/or burned out, quality and safety concerns will *never* be adequately addressed. It is impossible to disentangle the quality of care for the patient from the carer's professional quality of life; they are one. Health for the cared for and the carers is directly related to the care rendered and received; *how* we care transforms *our* professional quality of life (and our overall quality of life), and how patients receive care transforms their quality of living and dying.

Nurses, as transformers in health care, need that sense of oneness, that connectedness to other. We also need working environments that support the caring aspects that allow us to maintain and enhance our humanistic connection to those we care for and also those with whom we work. This caring connection is what enables most of us to discern meaning and purpose in our work and to be content at the end of the day.

THE FLAP OF A BUTTERFLY'S WINGS

Edward Lorenz (1993), a meteorologist, reiterated an old Chinese proverb when he asked, "Does the flap of a butterfly's wings in Brazil set off a tornado in Texas?" The answer is yes and no. We all know that subtle changes happen all the time. There are changes occurring that we are not even aware of; we are also not cognizant of the relationships among what seem to be different things. Chaos theory and new physical theories of the universe tell us that everything is irrevocably connected to everything else, they are inseparable, and we can rest assured that the flap of a butterfly's wings is contributing to change elsewhere in the world, although perhaps we will never quite know how or be able to quantify it. This incredible idea is called the butterfly effect (Lorenz, 1993), and it is relevant to any discussion on just about anything.

Nurses frequently do not recognize our enormous power. For many reasons, each of us might go through day-to-day work without ever being fully aware of how our actions contribute to transforming the lives of other people; we facilitate health and healing. We assist with life and living, dying and death. We *are* butterflies flapping our wings, so small and yet so powerful, seemingly insignificant and yet. . . . Did you know that the monarch butterfly manages to migrate thousands of miles each year back and forth from Canada and parts of North America to Mexico? It takes four generations of monarchs to manage this migration. It is definitely not a chance happening, although if one were to find a roost of monarchs (a large number of them resting together in a tree or bush) without knowing about their migratory pattern, one might just think, well how lovely, here is a bunch of butterflies. However, once one is aware of what the monarchs are doing, it takes on a very different meaning, does it not?

Some of you may know that the monarch migrates, and then it would not surprise you to come upon a roost of them. But what if you came upon a great many common buckeye butterflies? Would you think it was a chance happening? I can tell you that it is not; they too have a migratory pattern, although they are only heading south, not to Mexico. There is pattern and purpose in what they do, but what makes it even more amazing is that they have the ability—the power—to do it! It is a remarkable wonder of nature.

Many of us perceive our work and what we do as inconsequential, just so with a butterfly flapping its wings, but in actuality, what we do is momentous. It is not just a matter of what we do, but *how* we go about doing it that matters. If we are task oriented, for instance, focused on administering medications but not on the human-to-human connection part of our work, many of us will probably find that we feel less satisfied. Most patients will also tell us they are less satisfied with the care received when there is no person-to-person engagement. A thank-you note addressed to the staff on a unit is not for medication received; it is for *care* received. Meaningful are the words, thank you for *caring*.

Not too long ago I was asked to write something for a senior yearbook, and I shared the following story, trying to impart to the students the importance of cultivating and maintaining a connection with their patients. One day while I was speaking with one of the most influential bioethicists of our time, he shared his hospitalization experience with me. He said that some nurses were "chatty," while others "just went about doing their job," and that he repeatedly tried to engage several nurses in conversation, telling them about his work. He was so surprised that none of them showed any interest whatsoever in his life, who he is, or what he does. He wanted to know if this behavior (being distant) was the "norm" for nurses.

Upon hearing his comments, the thought that immediately came to my mind was that the nurses seem to have provided his care a bit *dispassionately*. Noticeably, he got the impression that his work was not important or impressive to the nurses who were caring for him. He was quick to say that he was not actually complaining about the care he received, but I certainly felt and relived his sense of disconnect and isolation as he spoke about it with me.

Unfortunately, I have witnessed, far too often and increasingly of late, the rendering of dispassionate care. We are facing a crisis in health care as we are being asked to do much more with much less, and consequently, it seems that many health care professionals (NOT just nurses!!) are suffering varying degrees of compassion fatigue or burnout. So, having been invited by the students to write for their yearbook, reflecting my take on pressing issues in nursing today, I reiterated something I have often said in various practice, supervisory, and educator roles over the years. Safe, competent practice is *not* the be all and end all of what nurses must do. Nurses should provide care not only with competence but also with compassion, otherwise one risks hindering, rather than enhancing, healing.

Briggs and Peat (1999) discuss "butterfly power" in their work on how chaos theory can inform and provide spiritual wisdom to those who pay attention to the underlying patterns of wholeness. Butterfly power means that whether we wish to or not, we are *always* part of whatever changes are occurring throughout the universe. We are participating, just by our very existence, and our participation is powerful. They noted the following:

> When we're negative or dishonest, this exerts a subtle influence on others, quite aside from any direct impact our behavior might have. Our attitude and being forms the climate others

live in, the atmosphere they breathe … If we're genuinely happy, positive, thoughtful, helpful, and honest, this subtly influences those around us. (p. 41)

Put the idea of positive subtle influence into the context of health care. It fits beautifully with many models that are based on the concept of "care."

NOTIONS OF GOOD: WHAT IT MEANS TO CARE

What does it mean to care? Caring is all about having a relationship with someone or something; it is about forming bonds between things, especially living things. You can care about your home but you are likely to care more about your husband, children, dog, or cat.

Many of our nursing frameworks and theories capture the essence of nursing and compassionate caring practices (see, Parker & Smith, 2010 and Fawcett, 2005, where a number of theories are detailed). While space does not permit discussing all of them, I want to briefly highlight how well our theorists have articulated the caring aspects of the science and art of nursing. The most prominent work on the nature of "care" has been written by nurse scholars Jean Watson (1988, 1999, 2008a), who developed a theory of human caring, also referred to as the theory of transpersonal caring, and Madeline Leininger (1984, 1994), who developed the theory of transcultural caring.

Leininger (1984) was one of the first in modern-day nursing to reflect upon, write about, and research *care* and caring practices in nursing. She noted that *"care is the essence and the central, unifying, and dominant domain to characterize nursing"* (p. 3) and went on to clarify the terms *care* and *caring*:

> *Care* in a generic sense refers to those assistive, supportive, or facilitative acts toward or for another individual or group with evident or anticipated needs to ameliorate or improve a human condition or lifeway.

> *Caring* refers to the direct (or indirect) nurturant and skillful activities, processes, and decisions related to assisting people in such a manner that reflects behavioral attitudes which are empathetic, supportive, compassionate, protective, succorant, educational, and others dependent upon the needs, problems, values, and goals of the individual or group being assisted. (p. 4)

Anyone familiar with Leininger's (1984, 1994) work knows that she emphasizes that although caring is a universal phenomenon, patterns of care can vary among cultures. A discussion on culture is not within the scope of this book; however, a notion of what it means to *care* is paramount to the discussion here; my own informal studies of how the majority of nurses respond to any discussion on human suffering and our own concurrent feelings of despair indicate that there is a subculture –a "nurseculture." We may not speak the same language and we may not all provide health care in the same manner, but we all feel compassion. As compassionate carers we, ourselves, are vulnerable to co-suffer with others and to become compassion fatigued.

In our line of work, caring makes all the difference. How one goes about providing care is paramount to healing; we always need to be cognizant of how we relate to others. There are two types of care in nursing: the instrumental, which refers to the technical and physical aspects of care, and the expressive, which relates to the psychosocial and emotional aspects (Woodward, 1997). In nursing, our ability to act in a compassionate manner entails using both kinds of caring. Hence, I intentionally use the word ca*rers*, rather than caregivers, because it seems to me that the word *carers* more effectively denotes who we are and what we do—not what we *give*; we do not just give care, we *care.*

Watson noted that "it is when we include caring and love in our work and in our life that we discover and affirm that nursing, like teaching, is more than just a job, it is also a life-giving and life-receiving career for a lifetime of growth and learning" (Watson & Woodward, 2010, p. 354). In her theory of human caring, she (2008a) describes the transformation that can arise within a single caring moment, a time when there is a deep connection between the person who is being cared for and the one who is the carer. Throughout her work, Watson emphasizes the important link between compassion for others and self, noting that when we bear witness to and ease the suffering of others, we are contributing to our own well-being and self-actualization.

Martha Rogers' (1970, 1992) nursing framework, the science of unitary human beings, formed the foundation for many other theoretic models, and while she did not overly stress compassionate caring, it was she who first conceptualized the idea in nursing that human beings and their environments are inseparable. What Rogers (1964) did point out in a little known book that she wrote on the importance of nursing, titled *Revielle in Nursing*, was that while nursing evolved as both a science and profession, "knowledgeable compassion replaces emotional naiveté" (p. 77). As women, and nurses, became more knowledgeable through erudition, they did not let go of their compassionate nature; instead, what had been perceived before as perhaps a weakness or naiveté, was noted to be a strength of our profession, when combined with higher education.

In 1964, many of Rogers' ideas were revolutionary; her advocacy for our profession a pulsing, vibrant voice:

Society's health demands that nursing stand firm in its conviction of its own social worth. Nursing alone is responsible for determining the core and boundaries of its education and services within the context of human needs and changing times . . . . The new tomorrow demands flexibility. Nurses must be able to adapt to the unknown. They must be receptive to new ideas and practices. They must reach out and grasp the unexpected with enthusiasm and with courage. Respect for human differences and for human endeavor must be a dominant value. (p. 92)

Rogers', description of nursing written in a New York University newsletter in 1966, clearly denotes nursing as both a science and art (Rogers, as cited by Malinski & Barrett, 1994, p. 338):

Nursing's story is a magnificent epic of service to humankind. It is about people: how they are born, and live and die; in health and in sickness; in joy and in sorrow. Its mission is the translation of knowledge into human service. Nursing is compassionate concern for human beings. It is the heart that understands and the hand that soothes. It is the intellect that synthesizes many learnings into meaningful administrations.

In Rosemarie Rizzo Parse's humanbecoming theory, nursing is all about enhancing quality of life and the nurse's *true presence* in bearing witness, being with and connecting to others during their living–dying experiences (Parse, 1994; Parse, 1998, 2007). Parse's development of this school of thought is noteworthy for its clear depiction of how we go about appreciating and caring for people. Meaning, rhythmicity, and transcendence, the major themes of humanbecoming, all get at universal wholeness, pattern, and transformational change (Parse, 2007).

From theorist Margaret Newman's (2008) perspective, nursing is about being fully present to explore with patients their evolving patterns of health exhibited by the process of expanding consciousness, which she defined as, "a process of becoming more of oneself, of finding greater meaning in life, and of reaching new heights of connectedness with other people and the world" (p. 6). It is through the nurse's relationship—our connection with others that consciousness expands—both for the patient and the nurse. It is a unitary process.

Another nurse scholar, Marlaine Smith (1999, 2010), noted converging ideas of caring in the work of Rogers, Watson, and Newman and developed a theory of unitary caring. She describes the phenomenon of unitary caring with five concepts: (1) manifesting our intentions (2) appreciating patterns, (3) attuning to dynamic flow, (4) experiencing the infinite, and (5) inviting creative emergence. Thus, we manifest our intention to assist with healing; we appreciate patterns of wholeness—oneness; we pay attention to our ways of being in the world; we acknowledge that this human-to-human connection is bigger than each of us separately—it is beyond us, it is sacred; and lastly, through our recognition of caring and our acts of caring we inspire ourselves and others "to birth oneself anew in the moment" (Smith, 2010, p. 499).

All models of care applied in practice are based on relationships and are sometimes referred to as relationship-based care, which is comprised of (a) the carer's relationship with patients and their loved ones, (b) the carer's relationship to self, and (c) the carer's relationship with coworkers (Koloroutis, 2004). No matter which model of care one looks at, the emphasis is really on the inseparable nature of the cared for and the carers.

Nursing, as a caring practice, has ethical comportment and notions of good embedded in our actions; as nurse scholar Patricia Benner (1994) wrote, it is "a way of knowing and not knowing" (p. 42). She suggested that, through our stories, the narratives of our experiences as nurses, we can gain a better understanding of the significance of our work. It is *care* that provides the foundation for a meaningful world; without it the world is meaningless— "nothing really matters" (p. 44). Yet, Benner also pointed out that "caring practices continue to be rather invisible, devalued, and typically inadequately accounted for in our institutional designs and public policy" (p. 43).

Benner (1994) pointed out that any professional practice "is a socially embedded organized activity with notions of good inherent in the practice and character of the practitioner" (p. 43). Without adequate recognition of *care* as an integral part of nursing practice, and undoubtedly, that it should be paramount in all health *care* professions, one chances its ultimate disappearance. Along this line of thought I am reminded of working on units where care acuity determined staffing and where viability (when the patient prognosis is good) was taken as indicative of higher acuity— which, in turn, equates with better staffing. To me, that always seemed a bit skewed. What of the family and friends of our patients, those people who were hoping for a cure, bearing witness to their loved one's suffering? Those people walking up and down the halls, sleeping in the waiting room, standing at the bedside, watching helplessly as their loved one slipped away. Why didn't they ever factor into the patient acuity level? How could they *not* be considered?

With an increasing emphasis on outcomes, there must be additional focus on the ways in which we in nursing work to make quality and safety come about and whether it meets our moral and personal standards. Florence Nightingale, as one of the most influential people of health care to date, emphasized quality and safety (and positive outcomes), but they were never the sole focus of her work.

Nurse scholar Margretta Madden Styles (1992) wrote of Nightingale's enduring symbolic representation of what it means to be a nurse:

> ... fragments pieced together form a collage of Nightingale as feminist, practitioner, politician, scientist, environmentalist, visionary reformer—a striking noble portrait. But I hold still another, a more personal, intimate picture in my mind.
>
> Displayed within a showcase at the entrance to our school is a letter written by Nightingale in 1855 to the parents of a young soldier who died of typhus in the Crimea. She describes his last moments. I fancy that she wrote it late at night fighting to overcome despair and fatigue, after she had finished her rounds with the lamp that, in turn, became her symbol. And I fancy that she wrote similar letters to the loved ones of all those for whom she cared so deeply and felt so profoundly responsible. (p. 75)

First and foremost for Nightingale, nursing was about compassionate caring for people. Her legacy lives on today in modern nursing. So why it is that many of us in nursing do not seem to know how essential our caring work is, how vital our unique contribution is to health care? How is it that we do not recognize our *own* importance? Whether intentional or not, it is in part the fault of our educational system and the systems in which we work where there continues to be demeaning and devaluing of the basic *caring* practices of nursing.

I am not laying the blame for this at anyone's feet; rather, I am asking for us to individually and collectively assume the responsibility. As a nurse and educator of nurses, I share some of my own mistakes and perceived failures quite honestly on these pages. I am certain that nurses who seem to be apathetic and dispassionate were *not* always that way. For why would individuals choose to come into a *caring* profession and then choose not to *care*? On units where care is dispassionately rendered and where healing often seems to be hindered rather than helped, it is clear that there is a collective wound. Staff and leaders who work in these areas are frequently fighting an uphill battle, perhaps sometimes even a losing battle.

FIGHTING AN UPHILL BATTLE

Taking a position as a clinical coordinator in a long-term care facility, I was assigned to cover an area that had a reputation for being the worst unit in the place. Some of the staff were not providing quality care.

It seemed they were *un*caring, and in a few instances, even abusive toward the patients, their families, and coworkers. I spent more sleepless nights while employed there than I have during my entire career. I lasted in that particular job less than a year.

I went to work dreading each day, and I went reluctantly home at night worrying about what I would find on returning the next day. I realized fairly quickly that I was hired to clean house and not only was this a difficult task, it was more than a little unpleasant. What kept me centered and able to do what was needed during the time I was employed there was my ever present focus on the well-being of those who were entrusted to our care. I recall how nurses and nursing assistants, who had themselves been seemingly battered for so long by their burnt-out coworkers and by the environment they were working in, seemed to rise to the task of assisting me to overcome some of the many obstacles that were preventing the rendering of compassionate, competent care. Still, the constant confrontations with difficult staff and union members finally wore me down; I could not sleep at all and my husband begged me to quit. Subsequently, I gave my 4-week notice and resigned.

Many of the staff were genuinely sorry to see me go and gave me a farewell party. I still have the plaque with the serenity prayer on it, given to me by a nurse who truly did care. You know, the one that begins with "God grant me the serenity to accept the things I cannot change ... ." It was very fitting, but at that time, I felt so guilty about having failed those people—both the residents and the staff. I remember thinking, I should stay and try to make things right.

Over the years, I have heard many stories like mine where colleagues were in staff or leadership positions that they had to leave. For some, the experiences they had were so unbearable that it prompted them to leave nursing entirely. For others, perhaps those who did not recognize the choices they may have had, the experience became a catalyst for illness or apathy or both. The stark reality is that the environments in which we work are not always conducive to health and healing for everyone, and it is not just a matter of insufficient staffing, which has always been perceived to be a big part of the problem. There is an increasing database of knowledge that indicates overall quality of care, clinical outcomes, and patient satisfaction are directly related to the workplace environment (Aiken, Clarke, Sloane, & Sochalski, 2001; Aiken, Clarke, Sloane, Sochalski, & Silber, 2002; Aiken et al., 2011), and we know that in poor work environments, there is a significantly higher incidence of nurse burnout and overall job dissatisfaction.

It is ironic that many of us in health care work in unhealthy environments where we are often forced to ignore our own needs and our own health—but for whom do we do this? Is it for the sake of the patient or the sake of the systems in which we are working? From the many years of Magnet (Drenkard, Wolf, & Morgan, 2011) studies in these United States, we know that a healthy workplace for us needs to be an inclusive patient-oriented care environment in which nurses are valued for what we contribute to the healing process on a multidimensional level, and where we are provided with the resources to do it in a way that leaves us feeling like we are doing our work well—where we can feel compassion contentment. The success of the Magnet initiative has shown us that we—nurses—are unquestionably the people who can and do make it happen. It is up to us to lead the effort to transform care. So, how can we do it? By remaining cognizant of the meaning and purpose of our work. How do we do it? With compassionate and competent caring, and perhaps with our code of ethics and Nightingale's (1859/1946) *Notes on Nursing* in our pockets.

KEY POINTS

- Everything is a manifestation of energy, purposefully transforming all the time.
- It is all essentially one, so whatever I do or you do is not just reflected in the whole; *it is the whole*.
- Subtle influences contribute to both positive and negative transformation.
- Nurses do not only provide care, we care. We are the primary transformers in health care for people during both living and dying.
- Health and healing for both the cared for and the carers is directly and simultaneously transformed by how *we*, individually and collectively, go to work each day.

Part 2

UNITY, PURPOSE, AND THE GOOD: AN ETHIC OF CARING

A human being is part of a whole, called by us the Universe . . . He experiences himself, his thoughts and feelings, as something separated from the rest—a kind of optical delusion of his consciousness. This delusion is a kind of prison for us . . . . Our task must be to free ourselves from this prison by widening our circles of compassion to embrace all living creatures and the whole of nature in its beauty.
—ALBERT EINSTEIN (1879–1955)

Chapter 3

COMPASSION AND CONTENTMENT: BEING HEARTFUL

*A commitment to kindness can be the thread that twines
throughout our various successes, disappointments, delights,
and traumas, making our lives seamless, giving us ballast
in a world of change, a reservoir of heartfulness to infuse
our choices, our relationships and our reactions.*
—SHARON SALZBERG

KEY TOPICS

- Compassion and compassionate caring
- Actualizing potentials as nurses
- Contentment
- Productivity and quality care

In the book, *Ruby's Imagine*, written by Kim Antieau (2008), Ruby, a teenager, lives in the heart of New Orleans in a small cottage with her grandmother. A hurricane, which Ruby refers to as The Big Spin, comes, and in its immediate aftermath, amidst terrible devastation and flooding, Ruby goes around the town in a raft with her friend Jay El and some others trying to help people:

> The day was so hot and humid and stinky that it was hard to breathe. We couldn't go fast because there was so much debris and tangled wires. We went to the first building we saw .... We helped one old man and woman, tiny and frail, step off their porch into our boat. They had a little dog about the size of a rat. He came too .... Next we got a family: a mother and her three tiny children. The mother couldn't stop crying. The babies

just look at her and us. I about start crying then too. The babies
didn't hardly have any clothes on them. I held the youngest one
on my lap close to me and said, "I'm sorry dawlin'. I loves you,
I loves you, I loves you." The baby rested her head on my
shoulder. (p. 140)

Ruby is a gem and the author's choice of a name is fitting. I have read this
book several times and I always get teary-eyed. Written in first person,
the portrayal is one of *compassionate caring* for others. Sharing her story
makes readers—us—more compassionate, for as we read, we recognize
in Ruby a generosity of spirit that always gets beyond herself, away
from her own pain and sorrow, to help others. We know it would be far
easier for Ruby to stay in a safe place and not bear witness to anyone
else's suffering.

COMPASSIONATE CARING—RUBIES, AND GEMS

In nursing, we rarely acknowledge that we too are rubies, like the student
who called Nurse Katie "a gem." Nursing is much more than physical
assessment, pathophysiology, pharmacology, and medical treatments.
Among my often-evoked memories of the many patients cared for over
the years, a male patient named Eddie comes to mind (Todaro-Franceschi,
2012). I encountered Eddie while working as a staff nurse in critical care.
He had been admitted to our cardiac intensive care unit with an inferior
wall myocardial infarction and was placed on several IV medications, an
arterial line and swan ganz were inserted, and oxygen therapy was started.
He was critically ill, but he was also alert and what everyone referred to
as difficult.

Over the course of several days, Eddie became outright belligerent.
He would pull on his lines while angrily telling us he did not want any
of it; all he wanted was to get out of bed. The physicians said he was becoming confused; the nursing staff, for the most part, agreed. A prescription
was written to use four-point restraints as needed. Placed in restraints,
Eddie began to be combative, pulling at his tubes and screaming to be
"let loose."

Nurses took turns going into his room and repositioning him, fixing
his lines, and trying to calm him down. Antianxiety medications were prescribed and administered. Not quite to the point of involuntary sedation
but looking very much like it was in his future, Eddie was still adamant
that he wanted out of bed, and finally, I asked him why. He answered, "I
don't want to die in a hospital bed all alone. I'd rather be sitting up in a
chair." I responded by saying that everyone was trying to help him get
better. He quieted down a bit while I moved around his room doing

all the things a nurse does. Then, he said to me, "I know I am dying." I didn't know how to respond to that at the time; it was years later that I learned a remark like that was an invitation—an opportunity to pull up a chair and be present with someone who is suffering, but his comment certainly got me thinking about ways we could perhaps better meet his needs.

All of us—the nurses, residents, and interns—discussed this patient's wishes with the attending physician when we made our rounds, after which we changed his activity level so that Eddie could get out of the bed to a chair. We procured a geri-chair, and when we got him into it, he was so grateful and pleased to have finally gotten through to us his basic need to get out of that bed. He remained out of bed, alert, and oriented, and he was a totally different person, no longer difficult or belligerent, no longer requiring restraints or antianxiety medication. At the end of that shift, we all felt pretty good with ourselves—the carers and the cared for. Our hearts were full. The patient was heartful because we had, like in the motion picture *Avatar*, finally been able to really "see him," and we were heartful because we recognized that we had gotten beyond ourselves and had actually "seen him."

This patient eventually did die on our unit, despite our attempts to save him. This wasn't surprising; many individuals have some foresight of their impending death. The eye-opener for me was that he was only comfortable and content when we stopped doing what *we* thought was most important (and admittedly the textbook picture) and instead listened and acknowledged his really small request to "allow" him to get out of the bed. We briefly turned our focus outward toward the whole of the person, rather than focusing on what seems in retrospect to have been *our* need and intent to *cure* the person, in a manner that we, and not the patient, believed was the right way to go about providing care. We moved beyond the rendering of competent care to compassionate care.

When nurses make choices and act on those choices as the intelligent, compassionate carers we are, when we are authentic and true to our purpose, it is clear that nursing is not just about following "orders" and ensuring that a proper medical regimen is followed. It is evident that our purpose is not solely about administering medications and measuring outcomes. Through our purposeful actions, we actualize our potential as nurses, assisting people to maximize their potential for health and healing in living and in dying. Herein we come to an ethic of care which emphasizes the foundation underlying our very being. We are connected, one *with* those we care for—and it is this unity and purpose that manifest the potential to heal.

In looking back at this case, I recognize now how fortunate all of us were to be on the same page; it could have been a battle between the few and the many, had anyone thought it was not clinically feasible to get the patient out of bed. I wonder, would I then have been courageous enough to fight that battle?

HAVING A SENSE OF "WE-NESS"

Compassion, a topic of great interest in both the Eastern and Western traditions, is considered to be a human emotion; however, it is also labeled a virtue, a good feature or desirable quality of people. The word *compassion* is taken from Latin, where it means to co-suffer. As with most aspects of human nature, it is always worthwhile to begin any discussion in this area by going back to the ancients. It is Aristotle (n.d./1984) who, through his conceptualization of "pity," is credited with the modern-day idea of "compassion." Pity is said to manifest as feelings of compassion for the suffering of others, and it can also be seen as a feeling of grief, mercy, or sorrow (Angeles, 1992). On the other hand, physician Larry Dossey (2007) emphasized that "compassion doesn't mean feeling sorry or pity for people but feeling with the other, learning to dethrone yourself from the centre of your world and put another there" (p. 1). Concern for others makes us selfless in a way; we are less likely to focus on ourselves. Consequently, compassion is not just something that one feels in relation to another's suffering; it is the experience of feeling *with* another (Blum, 1980).

Physician Eric Cassell (2005) stated that compassion "appears to be an emotion that is specifically social or communal, in the same family, perhaps, with the feeling of patriotism or group-specific feeling" (pp. 434–435). I like the term *communal* and use it frequently in my own work, since it gets at the inseparable nature of all things—the inextricable connection we have to everything else. Indeed, as Cassell pointed out, the core of compassion is connecting, and identifying, with others:

> ... the compassionate share the same universe with the sufferer—dark and light, air, gravity, noise, and quiet. Also shared are worlds of common values, ideas, beliefs and aesthetics. We know each other through proximity .... In other words we share community—a "we-ness" where all are joined .... (p. 441)

People differ in the intensity of their emotions, thus compassion varies; how one relates to and identifies with another will differ from person to person, as Cassell (2005) wrote: "What brings tears to the eyes of one is a matter of indifference to another" (p. 438). While this is surely the case, I believe that the majority of us who go into what are sometimes referred to as the "helping" professions do so as an act of compassion. It is our compassionate nature that provides the impetus for us to enter into service to begin with—for most, it is an impelled act.

Whereas many discussions on compassion emphasize the notion of co-suffering, I believe that suffering is not necessary, nor do we need to recognize it, if it is present, in order for us to feel compassion. It is an emotion and act of love. Compassion provokes action (need I say virtuous action?), which shows appreciation for something that seems outside oneself. It is knowing that something outside ourselves contributes to who we are and what we do. It is intuiting that whatever it is really *is not outside* of us at all.

Compassion Provokes Purposeful Action

In one of the most poignant articles on the importance of compassion, organizational behavior educator and researcher Peter Frost (1999) shared an experience he had in a hospital while being treated for cancer. He described witnessing the compassionate care of a nurse for a fellow human being who was suffering tremendously and who literally felt that he had come to the end of his life. Over the course of just one day, the nurse turned this patient's perspective so completely around that, later, the patient seemed like a different person. Frost, only an outside observer, was so moved by her compassionate actions that he claimed it changed the direction of his life. He began to study compassion in earnest, as a means by which organizations can be transformed. In his talks, published papers, and research, he repeatedly acknowledged the nurse. His witnessing of the compassionate care she provided to the other patient also later led him to write a letter commending her to the hospital administration.

I would bet that nurse was, and still is, not even partly aware of how significant her actions were that day. In that one instance, not only did she transform that patient's life, she changed Frost's life, and he, in turn, has transformed the lives of countless other people with his writings and research on compassion. There is no way of telling how many people have been motivated to change their behaviors and practices because of the purposeful actions of this *one* nurse with that *one* patient. Multiply that number by millions of nurses around the world and billions of purposeful actions over the course of our careers. WOW!

As I shared this story with a loved one, who recently underwent major surgery and came as close to death as one can come without dying, he tearfully recalled how, at a time when he felt himself slipping away, he heard one of his nurses keep saying to him, "stay with me, stay with me," and how the nurse had held his hand. He believes to this day that, without that act of compassion, he would have died.

Frost (1999) pointed out that one needs to have courage to act with compassion, for "one must often go beyond the technical, the imperative, the rules of organizations and beyond past practice—to invent new practices that have within them empathy and love and a readiness to connect to others" (p. 129). In nursing, to act with compassion frequently means fighting uphill battles; calling the physician 16 times to get scripts changed; calling the pharmacy for medications that have not come up; waiting for escort to take a patient down for a test for which the patient is NPO, or heck, taking a patient down for a test because escort isn't available and the patient is NPO! It might mean tweaking or blatantly ignoring the visiting hour policy for loved ones and getting into arguments with administrators over it. Or it could mean sitting in a patient's room when you really do not have the time for it, and then getting chewed out for "wasting" time, by coworkers who have lost their vision of what nursing is all about.

Nurse leaders are called upon to look at the things impacting on quality of care and to analyze all the factors to get at the source of a problem; in today's jargon, we call this "root cause analysis." We have always done this when looking at quality and safety issues. What we have not done consistently, and need to do, is spend more time exploring and appreciating the root cause of *heartfulness* in nursing, and then identify ways to foster and teach compassionate care. We need to explore more fully how we get contentment doing our work.

CONTENTMENT: A MATTER OF PURPOSEFULLY ACTUALIZING POTENTIAL

Most people spend the majority of the time, their entire lives actually, engaged in work. In essence, our professional quality of life *is* our quality of life, period. Consequently, everyone should begin each day, or at least the vast majority of our days, looking forward to going to work. Since we spend so much time at work, it should be a requirement that we be content or happy most of the time. That is a reasonable expectation, and yet so many people go to work and dislike what they do. But they keep doing it anyway.

When I began to think about writing this book, I was focused on two intertwining issues: (a) the quality of care being provided to patients who were very ill, perhaps dying, and their loved ones; and (b) the quality of the nurse's professional life. Little did I realize that I was really revisiting earlier works of mine. I mentioned my inquiry into ideas of energy in Chapter 2; in that work I was also led to explore ideas related to how people go about actualizing their potential (Todaro-Franceschi, 1998, 1999).

In trying to come to terms with what it means to actualize one's potentials in a purposeful way, I found that there was a general consensus among countless individuals who have studied human nature. The actualizing of human potential that manifests itself in happiness or contentment for people individually and collectively is directly related to an awareness and appreciation of things outside of ourselves and a perceived connection to other—other people and/or things (Todaro-Franceschi, 1998, 1999).

Whenever we use the terms *actuality* and *potentiality*, we are speaking the language of Aristotle. In fact, it was he who coined the term energy— *energeia*—and he defined it as both potential and actual things that are capable of change (Aristotle, n.d./1991; Aristotle, n.d./1996; Todaro-Franceschi, 1998, 1999). Aristotle also stressed that change comes about in a purposeful way. In his doctrine of four causes, he sought to answer the question of how and why a thing comes to exist—why there is a tendency on the part of things to actualize into whatever they eventually become.[1] Although he felt that things in nature have a tendency to become what they do, when it comes to the actualizing of human potential, Aristotle noted that there was always an element of choice; as rational beings we work by choice and not by necessity. Hence, according to Aristotle (n.d./1991, n.d./1996), everything has a purpose and *energeia*—when it becomes an actuality is a realization of that purpose. Purpose, generally speaking, implies meaning and intention, or a reason why something is being done. People are capable of actualizing potentials, and they do so in a purposeful, intentional manner.

When linked with happiness or contentment, the actualizing of human potential is frequently referred to as *self-actualization*. Self-actualization has been postulated as the one true motive for human existence (Goldstein, 1963). Psychologist Abraham Maslow (1968, 1971), who most readers are likely familiar with, explored the idea of self-actualization in depth, proposing a whole hierarchy of human needs, going from the most basic needs for survival—"safety and protection, to belongingness, love, respect, self-esteem, and identity"—and culminating, finally, in "self-actualization" (1971, p. 22).

Maslow (1971) defined self-actualizing people as individuals who are "without one single exception, involved in a cause outside their own skin, in something outside of themselves" (p. 43). Self-actualizing people tend to be happy, autonomous individuals. There is a long list of attributes for self-actualizing individuals, the most important of which is that they have an almost intuitive kind of feeling of *oneness with the rest of the world*. That feeling appears to motivate them into purposeful action.

In addition to feeling joyful or happy, creativity is another attribute that appears to exist in self-actualizing people. Maslow (1968) noted this characteristic and in his writings he referred to it not just as creativity in the usually depicted sense of art, music, writing, invention, and so forth, but also in very down-to-earth ways, such as "one woman, uneducated, poor, full time housewife and mother ... was a marvelous cook, mother, wife and homemaker" (p. 136). In nursing we have an overabundance of creativity. Consider the nurse who has a patient complaining of discomfort related to being bedridden and immobile, and as a result creates makeshift pillows to alleviate pressure points. Or the nurse leader who innovatively makes assignments because she is cognizant of her staff's strengths and weaknesses. And the nurse, Susie, in the story *Wit*, who hands her patient, Vivian, a popsicle and sits down beside her to eat the other half, while providing presence. All these nurses are creatively actualizing potentials in ways that help sustain their ability to do the difficult work they do, enabling them to remain connected to their work and the people in their environment and be able to provide quality care. The idea behind self-actualization is quite similar to Aristotle's (n.d/1984) notion of *eudaimonia:* "... happiness is an activity of the soul in accordance with complete excellence" (p. 1741),[2] where it is noted that "to be *eudaimon* is to flourish, to make a success of life" (Barnes, 1982, p. 78).[3]

Second Wind, Peak, and Optimal Experiences

So why is it that many people who work in health care do not appear to be happy? We choose to work in service to others, helping them to actualize their potential to heal and be healthy, to live a good life, and to die well; we should be happy or at least content most of the time. In an especially striking essay, "The Energies of Man," psychologist William James (1907/1987) discussed what he referred to as the phenomenon of *second wind*, the ability of human beings to go beyond their normal capabilities on various occasions. For instance, how is it that we can care for someone who is critically ill, stabilize that person after many, many hours, and leave work feeling wide awake and full of energy? Conversely, we can work an entire shift and, even though everyone has done fine, we may leave work feeling drained, disappointed somehow, bereft of that good feeling.

James (1907/1987) attributed the phenomenon of second wind to the idea that we have excess stores of energy that can be called upon as the need arises. He speculated that most of us rarely, if ever, tap our reserve store of energy. Still, by using our individual resources, we can actualize innate potentials—we can push ourselves to transcend feelings of fatigue without suffering any permanent, negative consequences. We sometimes go beyond what one could call the "normal" range of human ability.

Maslow (1971) wrote of *peak experiences*, wherein people feel extremely joyful, happy, or ecstatic. He noted that "any experience of real excellence, of real perfection, of any moving toward the perfect justice or toward perfect values tends to produce a peak experience" (p. 175). Peak experiences are similar to mystical experiences and meditative states, where one gets a sense that all is one. The person who has a peak experience displays many of the characteristics of the self-actualizing individual (Maslow, 1968, p. 97).

In a similar theory, psychologist and educator Mihaly Csikszentmihalyi (1990) detailed *optimal experiences* based on accounts of "how people felt
when they most enjoyed themselves" (p. 4). Optimal experiences occur
because one *makes* them happen: "The best moments usually occur when
a person's body or mind is stretched to its limits in a voluntary effort to
accomplish something difficult and worthwhile" (p. 3). Optimal and
peak experiences are both characterized by two important things: choice
and a sense of exhilaration or a feeling of accomplishment. By being in
control of one's actions and using conscious effort to meet preset goals,
one can experience great happiness.

Optimal experiences are based on the concept of *flow*. Csikszentmihalyi (1990) defined flow as, "the state in which people are so involved in an
activity that nothing else seems to matter; the experience itself is so enjoy-
able that people will do it even at great cost, for the sheer sake of doing it"
(p. 4). In order to be happy, we must *consciously* pursue the attainment of
goals: "Creating meaning involves bringing order into the contents of the
mind by integrating one's actions into a unified flow experience" (p. 216).

People can transform negative experiences into positive events if they
possess an *autotelic self*—"a self that has self-contained goals" (Csikszentmihalyi, 1990, p. 208). This means that we can take negative or potentially
negative things and transform them into challenges that we enjoy, and in
so doing, maintain a sense of meaning and purpose. When a person's
goals are threatened, Csikszentmihalyi noted that one can develop a "condition of inner disorder, or *psychic entropy*, a disorganization of the self that
impairs its effectiveness" (p. 37). Surely, from his stance, compassion
fatigue and burnout would be characterized as manifestations of psychic
entropy.

Csikszentmihalyi (1990) likened the human psyche to what are referred
to in science as dissipative structures, since the mind has the ability to turn
destructive events into positive ones.[4] He wrote of "transformational skills"
and the inherent ability people have to consciously unify experiences
toward the attainment of their goals: "Those who know how to transform
a hopeless situation into a flow activity that can be controlled will be able
to enjoy themselves, and emerge stronger from the ordeal" (p. 201). Can
you think of instances where things were wild on your unit, when it may
have been terribly short-staffed, and yet you still managed to make good
your intent to assist your patients with their healing? In all likelihood, the
cohesiveness of the health care team helped to make it happen. Everyone
being on the same page, with the same intent and purposeful effort, resulted
in feelings of contentment, despite the enormity of the workload.

We have optimal experiences because the intention is there—to do
something—to work purposively toward the actualization of some potentiality. In other writings, flow has come up as a powerful means of actualizing human potential to live fully and contentedly. Synchronicity or

meaningful coincidence, which I discuss in a later chapter, is also connected to flow—each builds on the other. Flow activities in nursing come about through purposeful, and often communal, actions in caring for others.

OPEN HEART, OPEN MIND

The Dalai Lama explains that in Buddhism, "the kind of love we advocate is love you can have even for someone who has done you harm" (Weber, 1986, p. 129). This reminds me of speaking with an Israeli nurse colleague, who shared her stories of caring for those who would (and sometimes did) kill her brethren, and yet, she was still able to feel compassion for those wounded soldiers. Being able to feel this way about those individuals who she considered enemies of her people surprised her. It is an unconditional love, born out of a sense that we are all one somehow.

Scholar Martha Nussbaum (1996, 2001) noted that the cognitive requirements of compassion hinge in part on the eudaimonistic philosophy of Aristotle. Intrinsic to the Aristotelian idea of human flourishing and happiness is a valuing of what it means to flourish and be happy (Nussbaum, 1996). For each of us, it means something different. Thus, in order to portray compassion, one must be able to empathize and identify with another; one must be able to picture himself or herself in the person's place. As she said, one must acknowledge that *this could be me*. Unfortunately, the acknowledgement that "this could be me" can sometimes lead to fear and distancing, if one isn't careful. This is where dispassionate care might replace compassionate care.

A nurse who is actualizing her potential as a carer is one who can feel compassion, who can put herself in the patient's place—repeatedly going to places that scare her. In some of the literature related to compassion, one comes across the word lovingkindness, used to denote an opening of the heart. This opening of the heart leads one to show kindness for another. It is sometimes associated with the Greek term *agape*, commonly used in Christian theology to refer to acts of kindness, motivated by love. It is love that impels us to care and to act with purpose, in essence, to show compassion.

In the Eastern philosophic tradition, there is a concept called *bodhichitta*, which is similar to the idea of compassion. Chodron (2001), explained that *bodhi* means "awake" or enlightened and *chitta* means both mind and heart or attitude (p. 4). The completely open heart and mind of bodhichitta can be equated with "the soft spot, a place as vulnerable and tender as an open wound" (p. 4). Human beings have a tendency to put up barriers to protect ourselves from feeling the pain of others, yet our bodhichitta—our soft spot—can overcome our fear of pain and suffering and instead allow us to embrace it.

Bodhichitta can be further described on two levels (Chodron, 2001). There is unconditional bodhichitta—"a just is" experience of "wow, this is good!" Then there is relative bodhichitta, which is of particular importance here, as Chodron notes this is the "ability to keep our hearts and minds open to suffering without shutting down" (p. 5). Kobat-Zinn (1994), when explaining mindfulness, noted the interchangeability of the words mind and heart noting, "... when we hear the word mindfulness, we have to inwardly also hear heartfulness" (p. 2). To be compassionate is to have an open heart and to be heartful. For nurses to be content at work we need to have both levels of bodhicitta, appreciating what is, and remaining open to our feelings of love and caring.

COMPASSION CONTENTMENT, PRODUCTIVITY, AND MAGNETISM: PEAS IN A POD

Work satisfaction comes about by meeting individual personal goals and feeling like we have accomplished something meaningful. When goals are set and met, this is referred to as productivity. In the case of nursing, work productivity basically means being able to provide quality care to our patients. But nurses are not in control of the multiplicity of things that feed into the provision of care. So can one be content or happy in the workplace but still feel dissatisfied? Conversely, might one be satisfied at work but still feel unhappy or discontent? I believe both are possible and that they are different constructs.

When I worked as a staff nurse on a medical unit, I would often be in charge and have 26 patients on a 52-bed unit. We would have no more than three nursing assistants working with us. At the end of our tour, none of us would leave on time, and I was frequently on the unit for an hour or more after the shift ended. Most nights I went home feeling content, knowing that I did everything I could to provide quality care. My patients felt cared for, often voicing their satisfaction. But was I satisfied? At the time, my salary was $18,500. I did not get paid any overtime and my husband was sure I was having an affair because I came home so late every night. I felt that none of the nursing staff were being acknowledged for the hard work we were doing and that we were expected to do far too much with far too little. I might have been content at the end of the day, but I was not satisfied with my work environment. My students who are out there in practice right now voice the same kinds of feelings; although they earn more money today, they are not satisfied. Why does this need to be a concern for everyone, especially nurse leaders? For starters, job satisfaction is one of the strongest predictors of an employee's intent to stay in a workplace (Böckerman & Ilmakunnas, 2008).

Jessica Pryce-Jones, cofounder of a British-based company that works with organizations around the world to enhance employee happiness, distinguishes between employee satisfaction and employee happiness. Pryce-Jones notes that the major difference between the two is control: "Satisfaction is determined by factors such as pay, working environment, and benefits. Happiness is a part of job satisfaction but really concerns what you can control and influence" (Scott, 2008, p. 9). What's more, she notes that "what people are in most control of is reaching their own potential" (p. 9).

According to Buerhaus (2008), we can expect that the reduced supply of, and increased demand for, nurses will lead to a shortage of 500,000 RNs by 2025. Shortages lead to heavier workloads, forcing higher nurse-to-patient ratios, which in turn affect nurse turnover and retention. All of this creates an environment that hinders, rather than promotes, the provision of quality patient care. Clearly, anything that contributes to an inability to provide the quality of care we want to give our patients will lead to work dissatisfaction, and over time, perhaps burnout, which then impacts the provision of care even more. It is a vicious cycle impacting the entire health care system and one that health care organizations are only just beginning to understand. Of all people, though, it is those of us in nursing who really need to understand this, because it is not just affecting our contentment at work and the quality of patient care that we are providing; it is much bigger than that. It is affecting us individually at work and at home, and collectively, as a profession. In addition, that butterfly effect goes out into the community of people that we serve and has increasingly become a societal issue as well.

From its inception, the Magnet hospital program rested on criteria that stressed the importance of the nurse in the creation and maintenance of a healthy work environment. Facilities that had a low turnover of nursing staff and seemed to attract nurses (like a magnet) were studied to identify what made them so attractive (McClure, 2011). Based on the findings of that original study several decades ago, at the onset, the Magnet model focused on the attraction and retention of nurses, nurses' job satisfaction, and quality patient care productivity (Drenkard, Wolf, & Morgan, 2011; Schmalenberg & Kramer, 2008). However, when these criteria were more closely explored by nurse researchers and others over time, it was found that up to 86% of attraction, retention, and job satisfaction was in fact related to the nurses' perceptions that they were providing quality care. Consequently, productivity became the main emphasis in the Magnet model.

In 2001, when nurses from 14 Magnet hospitals were asked what makes for a satisfying and productive work environment, they named eight main attributes: coworkers who are clinically competent, collaborative interdisciplinary relationships, autonomy in clinical decision making, supportive nurse leaders, personal control of nursing practice, support for education, a perception of adequate staffing, and a culture where concern for patients comes first (Schmalenberg & Kramer, 2008). It was noted that "a healthy work environment is a group-level phenomenon," and in health care organizations, this is especially so (Schmalenberg & Kramer, 2008, p. 66). Whether individuals perceive their work environment as conducive to their contentment is largely contingent upon how people interact with each other and how patient care is provided. Structural processes alone are not enough to render a happy workforce.

The modern Magnet model focuses on "proven outcomes" and has five components: transformational leadership; structural empowerment; exemplary professional practice; new knowledge, innovations, and improvements; and empirical outcomes (Wolf, Triolo, Reid-Ponte, Drenkard, & Moran, 2011). The first four all lead up to the last one, which is important in that it is understood that every single one of them are necessary components to the overall goal of providing quality care. Unfortunately, many places are so focused on outcomes that they cannot see the tree for the forest, and what happens is that they fall short of the mark. And who is often blamed? The nurse!

It might be that the Magnet model, which depicts empirical outcomes at the core, seems to highlight outcomes more, at the expense of all the others. Yet, that is clearly not its intent; it is meant to put the emphasis on all of the components that feed into change, and can transform outcomes from substandard to optimal. In order to get it all to work, we know that transformational leadership is necessary, and the main ingredients for transformational leadership include one having vision, along with influence, people skills, and clinical and leadership expertise. In nursing, we have many transformational leaders, but we have a lot more "would-be" transformational leaders. They "would be" transformational if they perceived themselves as having power. I would suggest that one's role or position does not preclude their ability to be a transformational leader and that, in fact, staff nurses can be transformational leaders, individually and collectively. I will return to this line of thinking a bit later (and often).

QUALITY CARE OR QUALITY CARING?

If we define quality care with work productivity or with outcomes, we fall short of the mark in each case. Nurses can be considered productive because we complete all of our nursing tasks within the time allocated, but we may not have been able to provide quality caring—compassionate care. We may have a positive outcome of care such as curing an infection, but we may not meet our own expectations of quality caring if, for example, the patient and/or family does not know how to prevent future occurrences of the infection because we did not have the time to sit with the patient and/ or family to discuss health care practices.

The quality of patient care is important to us—a necessary prerequisite for contentment. Inherent in quality care is quality *caring*. The nurse who can connect with her patients and not feel as if she is a robot is more likely to go home at the end of the day feeling heartful and more content.

Recently I went out in cyberspace seeking a few pictures to portray the idea of compassion for some work that I am doing. I went to a Creative Commons site to find pictures and did a search on the word "compassion." The pictures that came up to denote compassion were mostly of "doctors," "nurses," and "kittens." Obviously, it is believed to be an inherent characteristic of physicians and nurses that they are compassionate and that they emanate caring in their practice. One must ask, then, why many of us frequently find ourselves wondering about "that abrupt physician" or "that apathetic nurse." We find ourselves thinking, "something is wrong." Well, something *is* wrong. The bad and the ugly are taking the place of the good.

The crux of the matter is that attainment of happiness and contentment is achieved through the recognition of the interrelatedness of everyone and everything and our ability to appreciate it all as we go about our day-to-day nursing work. This knowledge encourages many of us to take purposeful action. One could say, then, that the actualizing of our potential as nurses is contingent upon feeling compassion for others—it is a requisite characteristic for *our* happiness, human flourishing, or contentment. Our sense of connectedness feeds our contentment as human beings and carers. Purposeful actions that foster and enhance our connectedness— our sense of we-ness—are the essence of nursing, and they are powerful in that they enhance the quality of living–dying for our patients, their loved ones, and for *us*, the carers.

When one recognizes that all things and people are inextricably connected, and that whatever one does transforms all else, it is presumed that one is more likely to act in ways that consider the whole. This, in turn, leads to acting with moral comportment. It is here that compassion becomes a virtue as well as an excellence and is valued as a requisite characteristic of the "good" nurse.

KEY POINTS

- Compassion is the ability to put oneself in another's place, and to "feel with" that person. It emerges from a sense of connection to others and other things and it provokes purposeful action.
- Actualizing our full potential as nurses entails acting purposefully and with compassion to assist in health and healing and, ultimately, to enhance the quality of living–dying for people.
- Compassionate caring is an act of love that facilitates feeling heartful. Happiness, human flourishing, or contentment for nurses arises from our caring practices.
- A healthy work environment does not emerge solely from quality care and positive outcomes; it is borne out of, and sustained by, *quality caring* for both the cared for and the carers.

ENDNOTES

1. Any "thing" is made of some stuff—this stuff without form is called the "material cause." In this stuff a change can occur. The pattern or form into which this stuff can be or is changed is called the "formal cause." The "efficient cause" is simply the thing that brings about change or initiates the activity whereby the change takes place. The purpose or reason for which the change takes place, "that for the sake of which," is called the "final cause" (See Aristotle, n.d./1991, n.d./1996).
2. Also see Aristotle's (n.d./1911) *Nichomachean Ethics*.
3. Aristotle's *eudaimonia* is an end, an actuality (*energeia*), toward which one strives.
4. Prigogine (1980) discovered that certain chemical reactions self-organize into complex patterns. Like chaos theory, the premise underlying this theory is that order can and does arise from disorder.

Chapter 4

VALUES AND EXCELLENCES IN NURSING

Morality means living with intentions that reflect our love and compassion for ourselves as well as our caring for others.
—SHARON SALZBERG

KEY TOPICS

- Code of ethics
- Compassionate care
- Commitment to self and others

E very profession has core values and excellences that provide an ethical code, a reference point for how we go about acting professionally. In nursing education, the learning of this content may be relegated to the clinical practicum experiences, and little time is spent on seminar discussions; thus, it often seems an obscure aspect of the curriculum. Yet, it is this more esoteric "stuff," which for me and many other nurse educators, has been, and continues to be, a challenge to teach to nursing students. Things like, for instance, how to question a prescription that does not seem necessary or correct (and the many other times when our advocacy is needed); bear witness to a dying person's anguish and comfort grieving loved ones; handle the bioethical issues you will face on an almost daily basis; remain connected to your patients while juggling the slew of tasks associated with your practice; and, of equal importance, how to care for yourselves and take the time to appreciate each day. It is the combination of a multitude of things (the whole!) that comprises the foundation for professional nursing practice, and all of it is so essential for both the cared for *and* the carer.

Introductory courses in nursing provide an overview of what professional practice is, what our code of ethics means, and how nurses are supposed to function. They usually outline the values and excellences held at the core of our being and becoming nurses. But very little time is allowed for dialogue and self-reflection. It is not enough to outline the values and excellences of nursing to those who are entering into the profession; each person must be able to reflect upon and understand how those values and excellences fit with their individual sets of values and beliefs, as well.

When I was growing up, I was told that children do not question their elders; they do as they are told. That dictate has never worked for adults. Of course, it is also no longer the case for children. Yet, here we are in nursing, teaching adults how to care for others, and in so doing, we briefly touch upon our professional code of ethics, but we never give our students time to question and truly understand those values. Instead, we emphasize the importance of quality and safety and skill sets such as assessment, wound care, medication administration, and the like, all the while taking for granted that the values and excellences emphasized in our professional code of ethics will be subsumed into our students' core through osmosis. It just does not happen that way.

OUR CODE OF ETHICS

I have had a bookmark from the American Nurses Association (ANA) since I graduated with my associate degree in 1982 that bullets 11 statements (referred to as provisions) of the Code for Nurses, dated 1976. Since then, the code has undergone two successive revisions, one in 1985 and again in 2001, and while the number of provisions has changed, the core elements have remained over time. That bookmark has traveled with me to various offices in places I've worked over the years. I continue to revisit it on a regular basis. It is a reminder of who we are and what we are individually and collectively always striving to attain. No one has captured the essence of our ethical code in a few words better than nurse ethicist Marsha Fowler (2008):

> Within the Code for Nurses, whatever the version, there is a deep and truly abiding concern for the social justice at every level; for the amelioration of the conditions that are the causes of disease, illness, and trauma; for the recognition of the worth and dignity of all with whom the nurse comes into contact; for the provision of high quality nursing care in accord with the standards and ideals of the profession; and for just treatment of the nurse. (p. xviii)

These words beautifully depict what the code is about, what *we* are about. And while the word compassion is not evident here, undoubtedly without it we would have no basis for any concern whatsoever.

COMPASSION: A VIRTUE AND AN EXCELLENCE

Compassion is unquestionably at the heart of the mission of the nursing profession; in our code of ethics, it is identified as both a *virtue* and an *excellence*. In the very first provision of our code, it is noted that "the nurse, in all professional relationships, practices with compassion and respect for the inherent dignity, worth, and uniqueness of every individual, unrestricted by considerations of social or economic status, personal attributes, or the nature of health problems" (Fowler, 2008, p. 143). It is made clear, in the interpretive statements regarding our code, that the use of the term "health problems" encompasses all aspects of human living–dying; both those who are well and those who are ill are the recipients of care.

The ANA specifically addresses the core values of the profession of nursing, noting that "excellences such as compassion, patience, and skill are habits of character of the morally good nurse" (Fowler, 2008, p. 161). We value compassion as a virtue—a requisite characteristic of the "morally good nurse," and we also acknowledge its function as an excellence—a compassionate carer does her work well. It is not enough to be able to do the technical skills of nursing competently. *Sine qua non*, both competent *and* compassionate care, have to be the basis for a nurse's work ethic; one without the other simply is not nursing.[1]

ALTRUISM: RENOUNCING NEEDS OF SELF, A MISNOMER

Nursing exists to serve society, as do all professions. Foundational to all professions is an ethic that is noted to be altruisitic, and in a way, we are expected to lay aside or renounce our own needs in order to do for others. Basically, altruism equals renunciation of the self. However, this is problematic because we cannot take care of others unless we are healthy and fit; we must first care for ourselves in order to be able to care for others. The best example that comes to mind are the instructions on an airplane: In the event of a loss of cabin pressure, oxygen masks will drop down and you are told that you need to apply the mask to yourself first, before you assist your children, loved ones, or others. There is an ANA provision in our code of ethics that shares a comparable message: "The nurse owes the same duties to self as to others, including the responsibility to preserve integrity and safety, to maintain competence, and to continue personal and professional growth" (Fowler, 2008, p. 158). We need to preserve our *own* well-being, caring for ourselves as we would care for others. In the biblical passage, we are told to do unto others as we would have them do unto us. In nursing, we need to realize this must go both ways; we must do unto ourselves as we would do unto others.

Preserving our integrity does not mean simply the physical aspects of our selves; it involves the psychological and spiritual parts of well-being. If we value caring for others and it is the impetus behind our work as nurses, then by our purposeful acts of caring for others we are also caring for ourselves. Conversely, by not doing so, we are hurting ourselves. Obviously, then, if nurses are to do for ourselves, we must be true to our authentic selves; we must always remember our purpose.

PRESENCE AND AUTHENTICITY

Bishop and Scudder (1996) discussed what it means to have a therapeutic caring presence, showing the relationship between compassion and authenticity. They note that a good nurse is one who is not only competent but is also obviously concerned with the well-being of those she is caring for. A caring presence,

> is a way of being with others that assures them of personal concern for their well-being. This way of being fosters trust, mutual concern, and positive attitudes that promote good health. When caring presence pervades a health care setting, the whole atmosphere of that setting is transformed ... (p. 41)

A good nurse may also be referred to as an "exemplary nurse," someone who "did their work in a remarkable way and achieved outstanding outcomes for their patients and, subsequently, were positively affected themselves" (Perry, 2008, p. 88). In Perry's study of exemplary oncology nurses who seemed to avoid compassion fatigue, she found several common themes: moments of connection, making moments matter, and energizing moments, which all refer to caring practices (p. 87). Notably, the new Magnet model emphasizes the notion of "exemplary nurses" and links it to both job satisfaction and positive clinical outcomes. What needs to be stressed more is that when we do our work well, we feel good, yes, but a main part of nursing work is the human-to-human connection that takes place: "The precursor to caring is connecting" (Clayton, Murray, Horner, & Greene, 1991, p. 155).

Why do people choose to go into nursing? In one of her early works, Watson (1985) identified that "human caring is the moral ideal and origin for nursing's professional role and 'calling,' with the goal of protection, enhancement, and preservation of human dignity" (p. 74).

I believe that the vast majority of people who choose to enter into nursing do so because they feel compelled to care; they have an affinity for the work. It may not always be that nursing was their calling, but that caring for others in some manner is their calling.

In his writing on the attributes of a profession, Ernest Greenwood (1982) emphasized that "professional work is never viewed solely as a means to an end; it is the end itself. Curing the ill, educating the young, advancing science are values in themselves" (p. 30). He noted that there is devotion to the work; so much so, that on occasion, the "work-life invades the after-work life, and the sharp demarcation between the work hours and the leisure hours disappears" (p. 30). I am reminded here of Maslow's (1968) notes from his studies of the self-actualizing individual: "Duty became pleasure, and pleasure merged with duty. The distinction between work and play became shadowy. How could selfish hedonism be opposed to altruism, when altruism became selfishly pleasurable?" (p. 140). The bottom line is that professionals who exist to serve society also serve themselves in that they so enjoy (*or should enjoy*) what they do that their altruistic nature is not really a renunciation of self—rather, it is an embracing of one's authentic self.

DOCTOR'S ORDERS

So here we have a nursing workforce that has an affinity for the work and wants to help people actualize their potential for health and healing. BUT the system will not let us do it, right? One must ask, is it the system that gets in our way, or is it us? I believe that it is neither alone; it is a combination of both.

Nurses are still predominantly socialized during basic education and in the workplace to be subordinate to others. This is not always intentional; rather, it seems that old habits die hard. For example, when teaching pharmacology to baccalaureate students, I always emphasize that nurses do not "take orders" from others but are responsible for our actions. One of the ways I try to brainwash students is by telling them on the first day of class that every time I say the phrase "doctor's orders," they are to raise their hands, and the first five or so students to do so will receive extra credit on their lowest exam grades. This worked superbly although, one day, a student told me how angry another faculty member had gotten when all the students raised their hands every time she said "doctor's orders" during her lectures. I just laughed and said I would speak with my colleague. It was fine; when I did speak with her, we laughed together.

The following year, when I had this same cohort of students for a senior-level preceptored practicum, I noticed that many of them actually used the term "doctor's orders," themselves, in their speaking and writing. When I think of this, I cannot help echoing nurse ethicist and educator Joan

Liaschenko's (2008) words, "I no longer know what nursing academia is doing—the logic escapes me. I wonder what identities are being produced and against which nurses will evaluate themselves" (p. 201). She asked, "What moral resources is academia providing?" (p. 201).

Liaschenko (2008) noted that the current day-to-day experiences of nurses in practice are alarmingly similar to those of practicing nurses from years ago (when she began nursing school in 1967). Her own experiences in practice from 1970 through 1996, along with the stories she has continued to hear from her nursing students, reflect that the moral concerns of students mirror those of practicing nurses in the way they center on the conflict between themselves and others who are involved in the care of patients. Unsurprisingly, the majority of their shared concerns involved end-of-life care issues and/or times when a patient was critically ill. During these times, conflict often arose when other members of the health care team were not hearing the voice of the nurse.

What leads Liaschenko (2008) to question the logic of academia is that her graduate nursing students continue to question their own abilities and blame themselves for not being heard. She reflected that:

> ... students frequently wrote that they should have known more, the implication being that if they did, they would have been able to convince the physician to alter the course of clinical actions. The knowledge they feel they should have known was always scientific. (p. 196)

She goes on to note that "nurses fail to claim credit for their nonscientific knowledge that is absolutely necessary for patient care" (p. 198). Like Liaschenko, I believe that this is in large part due to the way we continue to educate nurses.

Going back to "doctor's orders," some readers may think, well, after all that is what they are called in practice; yes, but, we all know that *"orders"* are not what they really are. Nurses are responsible first and foremost to those we serve—our patients and their loved ones—and not to those who work beside us. Accountability goes in both directions; the nurse is accountable to the physician and other members of the health care team concerning the provision of quality care to people who need it. The physicians and other health care professionals, including administrative personnel, are also accountable, to us—nurses. Yet, somehow, many nurses do not get that message in their basic nursing education, or if they do, many of them seem to be quickly socialized "out" of it.

One year, a very upset student shared with us in class a sign that she had seen posted on a nurse's locker door by an administrator. I do not recall the exact wording, but it said something along the lines of, "I will not change or question doctor's orders." She was being publicly flogged! Back then, and *then* is only about 5 years ago, all I could think of were the words in the New York State Nurse Practice Act that said we should not vary an existing medical regimen.

I recently revisited the New York State Nurse Practice Act, which is posted online, and in 2012 it still says this: "A nursing regimen shall be consistent with and shall not vary any existing medical regimen" (see http://www.op.nysed.gov/prof/nurse/article139.htm). One must question the logic of that statement if we are indeed to uphold the basic premises of our code of ethics through our actions. How can we purposefully act with moral comportment and courage if we think that we are subordinate? How will we ever move away from this archaic view if our formal nursing education reinforces this way of thinking?

Questioning "Orders"

I had assigned one of my senior baccalaureate students to work with a patient named Joe, who had a primary diagnosis of colorectal cancer (Todaro-Franceschi, 2010). Joe had been admitted for further diagnostic testing, and just the day before, it had been discovered that he had widespread metastasis. He was alert, oriented, and conversant. The first day of our clinical rotation, he was walking with minimal assistance and verbalized feeling very little pain; MS Contin was effectively controlling any discomfort. The second day, in the early morning, I saw the student by the nurse's station around the time that breakfast trays were being delivered to the unit. I inquired about Joe and she informed me that he was still asleep. I asked about his vital signs and all the other normal things that an instructor might ask, like whether he was easily awakened, how his skin color looked, and so forth. As we walked to the patient's room, she assured me that he was okay.

At the patient's bedside, we found that his breakfast tray had been set up in front of him. Although he was in a semi-Fowler's position, Joe was fast asleep, his food untouched. Leaning in, I gently nudged his arm, while asking him if he wanted to eat his breakfast. With obvious effort he responded to me, opening his eyes slowly and saying, "yes, I am hungry . . ." and without completing the sentence, he was again asleep. After several attempts to speak with Joe, during which time he said he "just couldn't keep his eyes open," I asked the student to get his medication record. We found that at 6 p.m. the evening before, a fentanyl (Duragesic) patch had been applied for pain management. A potent opioid-derivative narcotic, fentanyl skin patches are very effective pain relievers; however, in Joe's case, the medication was sedating him.

Further exploration revealed that although Joe had requested pain medication in the late afternoon the previous day, his requests for pain relief had been infrequent during his 5-day hospitalization. Thus, the use of pain medication, which resulted in Joe's sedation, seemed extraordinary rather than ordinary care, and prompted many questions. Was the health care provider (HCP) who had prescribed the medication aware that Joe was being sedated with its use? Was it really necessary to sedate Joe to manage his pain? Was pain management along with sedation the intended outcome of the medical treatment? More importantly, what were this patient's wishes regarding what was to be *his* "dying" experience?

The nurse assigned to Joe that day had floated to the unit and was not familiar with Joe; she felt uncomfortable calling the physician to question the prescription for the fentanyl patch. I offered to make the call and spoke with the physician who had prescribed the medication. He informed us that Joe had been adamant that he did not want to have any pain. But, I wondered aloud, did the patient want to sleep the rest of his life away? I noted that he could not even stay awake long enough to eat his breakfast. The physician did not answer that question and instead indicated his irritation with my questioning his "orders." After a brief discussion with the primary nurse, the student and I went back into Joe's room, removed the fentanyl patch from his arm, and I asked the student to pull up a chair to wait for the patient to fully awaken, at which time she was instructed to inform me.

Later in the day, when Joe was awake and after he had eaten, the student and I sat down to speak with him. I asked him what he knew about his illness and he told us, "Well now, I'm dying." He explained to us that his cancer had spread, and that they—the doctors—could not get rid of it. I proceeded to ask him if he was currently in a lot of pain. Joe informed us that he was not in much pain and a wonderful discussion ensued during which time Joe shared a lot of things with us: He had been a widower for several years and he had two daughters who lived in Florida but were currently up North to see him. He told us that both of his daughters were insisting that he move to Florida to live with them, but because he did not want to be a "burden" to his children, he had not entertained the thought of relocating.

We discussed his living–dying options at some length and then I went to the nurse manager of the unit where we planned a meeting for Joe and his family, with the physician, nurse manager, and case social worker, the following day. Ultimately, Joe chose to move to Florida with his daughters, where hospice services were put into place.

There are several practice issues here that are directly related to compassionate caring and the concomitant moral comportment with which nurses go about our purposeful actions. In this case, the purpose of the pain medication that had been prescribed was to alleviate suffering, but it was not meant to sedate the patient. Had "doctor's orders" been followed, rather than questioned, and had we not taken the initiative to remove the patch, it would have remained on Joe and he would have been left to sleep. In all due likelihood, Joe's daughters would have thought his sleeping was due to the natural progression of his illness.

Had the nurse, who was caring for the patient that day, and the prescribing physician, put themselves for a moment in the place of either Joe or his family, they probably would have taken a different approach to his pain management; in other words, their purposeful actions would likely have been more compassionate and morally sound. The significance of the issues related to the physician's practice is beyond the scope of this book; however, the issues related to the nurse's practice must be more fully explored.

It is difficult to float to a unit where one is not familiar with the patients and the staff; I know this because I worked full time in the float pool of a 600-bed hospital for 2 years. Still, had I been in that nurse's shoes, I would have picked up the phone to call the physician. This is not because I am a better nurse, but because I have always been able to put myself in the place of the patient. I co-suffer well. I also know that somehow I did get the message early on in my professional career that without *us*, the system does not work at all. In addition, and perhaps most important here, is that I have always felt *free* to be moral. I have always believed that because I am a licensed registered nurse, my practice is autonomous—I answer to myself and my patients. Sadly, many nurses do not feel free to be moral.

Nursing practice must be collaborative, yes, but ultimately, it is autonomous in nature; the morally good nurse should intuit that she is free to act always in the best interest of her patients and their loved ones. Going back to Joe and to the float nurse, had she called the physician and questioned the medication, what would have been the worst-case scenario? I am sure the physician would have said the same things to her that he said to me. Had she pulled the patch off and sat down to speak with Joe, he would have shared the same things with her that he shared with the student and I. The outcome would have been the same; however, I would be telling the story from the nurse's voice instead of my own. It would have been *her* story.

I have no idea if the nurse who floated to the unit that day ever went back to the unit and became aware of the outcome for Joe. I do know that I feel *heartful* every time I recall how we were able to act purposefully to help him. Compassion is a virtue and an excellence that makes all the difference. How many family memories would have been lost had Joe been allowed to sleep through that day and the days thereafter?

VALUING COMPASSION AS A REQUISITE CHARACTERISTIC

While we spend very little time speaking directly about it in nursing education, as previously noted, compassion is a requisite characteristic for those who enter into the health *care* professions. Nurse educator Maria

Schantz (2007) claimed that the meaning of the concept *compassion* has not been adequately defined in nursing, and it is not widely promoted or emphasized in contemporary nursing practice. In a concept analysis, she detailed the differences among terms we commonly use in nursing, such as *empathy* ("a vicarious participation in other people's emotions, ideas, or opinions"), *caring* ("a state of mind, which is related to troublesome worries, anxiety, or concern"), and *sympathy* ("an overall kinship with someone's feelings, regardless of the feeling"; p. 51). Schantz noted that although these terms are related to compassion, compassion is the only one that "impels and empowers people to not only acknowledge, but also act toward alleviating or removing another's suffering or pain" (p. 51). And, in this connotation, lies a clear demarcation between the idea of compassion as an emotion—a feeling, versus the idea of it being a virtue and an excellence. It is in our *purposeful actions* to assist in healing that the characteristic of compassion as both a virtue and excellence becomes prominent.

In a recent concept analysis of *compassionate care*, repeating themes were identified in the literature, which seem to be the prevalent characteristics (of compassionate care) (Burnell, 2009):

a. A dimension of caring,

b. Sympathetic consciousness of another's distress,

c. Sensitivity to the pain and brokenness of another,

d. Suffering alongside another,

e. A spiritual connection with another person,

f. Attempting to comfort or alleviate the suffering, and

g. A demonstration of the fruit of the Holy Spirit.[2] (Burnell, 2009, p. 321)

To be a compassionate nurse essentially means that we feel for others, display kindness to others, and act on behalf of others for their benefit. We have an awareness of the interconnected nature of everyone and everything; it is all essentially one (Todaro-Franceschi, 1999). So, when someone is distressed, a compassionate carer acknowledges and bears witness to that suffering and will seek to lessen if not completely obliterate that anguish. Compassionate carers are concerned for the well-being of those entrusted to their care *and* will also willingly acknowledge that the significant others of our patients are also entrusted to our care (for they are suffering with, and sometimes more than, their loved ones). Yet, a compassionate carer also intuits that, by caring for others, we are also caring for ourselves; it is virtually indistinguishable where one ends and the other begins.

KEY POINTS

- Compassion is both a value and an excellence in nursing.
- Competent and compassionate care is the basis for our work ethic; one without the other is not nursing.
- By serving others compassionately, we serve ourselves and are authentic to our altruistic nature.
- Acting purposefully with moral comportment and courage entails being accountable to ourselves and expecting accountability from other members of the health care team. Thus, there is no such thing as "doctor's orders."
- Valuing compassion as a requisite characteristic for the profession means we need to embrace our compassionate caring practices and foster caring for self and other. We must do unto ourselves as we would do unto others.
- It is all one.

ENDNOTES

1. One could make an argument that overall competency in nursing practice must include compassion.
2. This, Burnell 2009 noted, is a biblical reference to nine attributes: "love, joy, peace, longsuffering, gentleness, goodness, faith, meekness, and temperance" (p. 321). Burnell identified these visible attributes to be significant as they "embody the heart of compassionate care" (p. 321).

Chapter 5

THE *ART* OF REAFFIRMING PURPOSE

> *So many people walk around with a meaningless life. They seem*
> *half asleep, even when they are busy doing things they think*
> *are important. This is because they're chasing the wrong things.*
> *The way you get meaning into your life is to devote yourself to*
> *creating something that gives you purpose and meaning.*
> —MORRIE SCHWARTZ

KEY TOPIC

- *ART*: A Model to Enhance Professional Quality of Life

When caring work becomes just work, and one is dreading going to work each day, it is time to *Acknowledge* that there is a problem. It is time to *Recognize* and explore one's options, reexamine intentions, and reaffirm purpose. And, it is time to *Turn* outward, to focus on self and other.

What nurses need is to have a practice that emulates connection with ourselves and with others. Most of us start out that way. Like children are more aware of their connection to things, the majority of us, as nursing students, are very aware of the human-to-human connection. Later on in school, students are taught to distance themselves, to apply a "therapeutic use of self," and they are essentially told to be empathetic while always remaining objective. This kind of classic teaching may inadvertently set the stage for the development of burnout later on; disturbingly, some nurse researchers have reported findings that suggest that the nursing educational process may lead to a reduction in caring behaviors (Murphy, Jones, Edwards, James, & Mayer, 2009).

The reduction of caring behaviors, by whatever means, brings us further away from compassion contentment because it encourages disconnection and distancing rather than connection and presencing. Still,

I remain convinced that nurses know more than most that "everyone needs to feel a sense of belonging, in living, and in dying" (Todaro-Franceschi, 1999, p. 130). Watson (2008b) emphasizes that we need to consider an ethic of "belonging before being" (p. 304). This ethic, I believe, has been the light that propels most of us to choose a nursing vocation; however, somewhere along the way, many nurses seem to forget our reason for *being* what we are. We deny that sense of connection to other. The nature of the health care system contributes to this sense of disconnect, and it often prevents us from remembering the reason for our *being* during our day-to-day living-working.

Years ago, when I recognized that many RNs who were coming back to school were not content with their work, I began to incorporate this knowledge into many of my classes. In an elective offering I wrote and regularly teach, I do a lot of work trying to bring compassion contentment back into the nursing practice of my RN to BSN pathway students. The course is about changing death experiences in health care, however, teaching this content for so many years has taught me the profound applicability of Virginia Woolf's words when she wrote, "I meant to write about death, only life came breaking in as usual" (Woolf, 1922). No discourse on dying and death is very meaningful without equal attention to life and living.

I begin the course by telling the students that they are there for a reason and that no matter what brought them to enroll in the course, their lives will be forever changed by the end of the term. At the end of the course I ask them to identify one AHA!, a moment where things seemed to come together to make more sense for them. The majority of the students share more than one, and sometimes many, AHA! moments like the following one written by an RN to BSN pathway student:

> *My second AHA! moment happened when one more time I got inside myself and I was able to reflect on the real me. That was when we spoke in class about finding some time in our busy work schedule to pull up a chair and talk with our patients. After this class, I realized how much I have changed since I became a nurse—to tell the truth, for the worse . . . . I still remember how passionate I was about my work, how very eager I was to stay one or two hours after work to finish documentation for which I never had time during my normal work hours because I had chosen to spend all this time with my patients. Many times I was ridiculed by other nurses and was told that I had a problem with time management . . . . I also recall my conversation with one of my coworkers who asked me why I like to work on Medical-Surgical units and not in the Emergency Department. I told him that I really enjoy talking with my patients and I don't have time when working in such a busy place as the ER, where you work like a robot that only follows orders.*

*After taking this class, I realized that working for $2\frac{1}{2}$ years as a floater
on many different units has changed me a lot. Now I am no longer
willing to stay after my regular work hours, no longer am I getting
into long conversations with my patients, and the place that I like
the most is . . . . Emergency Department, the place where I became
one of those robots . . . . Am I happy with who I have become? I am
not sure about it. But I am certain about one thing—I am glad that
I have taken this class because it has opened my eyes to myself; I am
more aware of myself, my unresolved conflicts, my hidden angriness,
my current preferences and who I am right now . . . .*

Nurses need to reawaken what most of us intuited when we first
entered into nursing—that it is all essentially one. We need to reaffirm a
sense of both unity and purpose. What is deemed negative or bad—compassion fatigue—is a pattern of the whole, a pattern which indicates that
transformation is needed. When we get to the ugly—burnout—we have
become automated, apathetic, and are working mindlessly rather than
mindfully.

WHAT PURPOSE?

Some of you may be asking yourselves, is there a purpose in the things I
do as a nurse these days? You may be wondering exactly what it is that I
am referring to when I write of reaffirming purpose. You might think, "I
am running around for 12 hours, with barely a moment to myself; it
seems all I do is administer medications and check prescriptions for accuracy. In between I document, and document, and document. Occasionally
I empty a bed pan, or turn a patient, but most of the time the only interaction I have with my patients is when I am giving meds. I might speak
collegially with a physician or therapist, but more often than not I feel
like I am being spoken *to* and not *with*. Increasingly, of late, I find myself
avoiding having to speak with patients and their family members;
who has time for them and what can I say to them that will make any difference, anyway?"

Does any of this sound familiar to you? If so, then you are right to question what I mean by *our purpose* in nursing, and most assuredly, you need
help to recognize and reaffirm your sense of purpose. It is not easy, and I
will not claim that anything *will* be fixed; I only claim that it *can* be fixed
and that each of us always has a choice in how we go about being in the
world, both personally and professionally.

What I mean by reaffirming purpose is that nurses who have forgotten
or lost enthusiasm for nursing *can* recover zeal (or ardor?) for who we are
and what we do. Individually and collectively, we can heal from and/or

possibly avert compassion fatigue or burnout, and at the same time, reaffirm purpose in nursing, by following certain steps depicted by the acronym *ART*.

ART: A MODEL FOR ENHANCING PROFESSIONAL QUALITY OF LIFE

ART entails *A*cknowledging, *R*ecognizing, and *T*urning Outward. Over the years, as I have taught and presented on this topic, I have come to think of the *ART* of reaffirming purpose as a healing model for our wounded work-force (Todaro-Franceschi, 2008). Following these steps can help you enhance your professional quality of life.

You first need to *acknowledge* your feelings and that you may have wounds, wounds that you have not been aware of and that are festering. With this newfound knowledge, *recognize* the choices that you have and reexamine your intentions. Then, through your purposeful actions based on the choices you make, you can *re-enchant* yourself with the nature of your work. Lastly, you must *turn outward* toward yourself and others. It is through reconnection rather than *dis*connection that we can prevent and/or overcome feelings of compassion fatigue and burnout. In Auden's classic 1940 poem, he notes we must "love each other or die." We must love ourselves as we love others too. In health care, it is through our connection to self as well as other that we can maintain and enhance our individual and collective professional quality of life; I call this my *reconnect contention*. Understanding and practicing mindful aware-ness (also referred to as mindfulness practice or meditation) can broaden your ability and make it easier to use *ART*.

Mindful Awareness

Mindful awareness is an ancient Buddhist practice that can be acquired through study. It denotes a way of being connected with the rest of the world by making a conscious effort to do so. Mindful awareness really entails *being aware of being* and doing it while you are in the moment. Some people might get turned off when they hear it is a form of meditation, but it is not the kind of meditation that requires one to drop everything. It is actually more like embracing everything, by being attentive and aware of it. Accepting it, just as it is.

I became enamored with mindful awareness in 2003 when I was diag-nosed with uterine cancer and one of my daughters bought me an audio-tape of the book, *Wherever You Go There You Are: Mindfulness Meditation in Everyday Life* (Kabat-Zinn, 1994). Although I had a vague idea of what it was, I had never practiced mindful awareness. It was fitting at the time that I learn the lesson that mindfulness meditation expert Jon Kabat-Zinn was teaching. When I was diagnosed with cancer, I became worried about the future, about having surgery, surviving surgery, developing complications from surgery, learning I might have advanced cancer, and ultimately, I was worried about dying and what would happen to my family. I was so fixated on what *might* happen that I could not appreciate what *was* happening, right there in each moment. Consequently, I was losing all of my moments.

Mindful awareness helps one appreciate the present, and as Kabat-Zinn (1994) noted, the present is really all we have; what is past already happened, but what is happening right now will transform our future. In light of that he asks, should we not pay more attention to our *now?*

> In every moment, we find ourselves at the crossroad of here and now. But when the cloud of forgetfulness over where we are now sets in, in that very moment we get lost ... . By lost, I mean that we momentarily lose touch with ourselves and with the full extent of our possibilities. Instead, we fall into a robotlike way of seeing and thinking and doing ... . If we are not careful, those clouded moments can stretch out and become most of our lives. (Kabat-Zinn, 1994, p. xiii)

Who has not, at one time or another, gotten caught up in a robotic way of being? It is, as Kabat-Zinn (1994) noted, our nature to be habitually unaware as we go about our lives.

Mindful awareness stops the mechanical activity of the mind, because once you are aware of what you are doing, you are "thinking" about the moment you are in, rather than unthinkingly acting. When applying *ART*, being mindfully aware will help you to complete each step of the process. In the following chapters, I often encourage you to be mindfully aware of your feelings and thoughts; you will be prompted to "capture your moments" (Kabat-Zinn, 1994, p. 17).

Step 1: Acknowledgment

Acknowledgment of our feelings is accomplished by self-reflection and mindful awareness. How do you feel, right now, in this moment? If you are reading this book, chances are that you are already unhappy with your work and are searching for ways to improve your professional quality of life. Or perhaps you are a nurse leader and are searching for ways to increase staff retention or help them improve productivity. Acknowledging that there is a problem and identifying what is contributing to it involves looking back and trying to discover turning points, accompanied by in the moment reflection on one's current experiences and behavior.

Narrative storytelling is a useful way to identify turning points. In some instances, it may also entail exploring the behavior and experiences of others who are sharing or have shared your moments. As you go about your work, try to look toward yourself, your actions and reactions to others, coworkers, patients, and the environment. Jot down your thoughts and feelings. Identify patterns of behavior and any negativity. Has the way you go about your practice changed for the better or worse since you began nursing? If so, can you identify when it started to change?

The Dalai Lama emphasizes that "If you directly confront your suffering, you will be in a better position to appreciate the depth and nature of the problem" (Dalai Lama & Cutler, 1998, p. 136). The problem with us in nursing is we often do not realize we are suffering. We have to learn how to be mindfully aware, as Madeline Ko-I Bastis (2000) shared with us how she learned to "sit in the midst of my suffering, feeling my feelings" (p. xiv).

There is this great little book written by Kent Keith (2003) titled, *Do It Anyway: The Handbook for Finding Personal Meaning and Deep Happiness in a Crazy World*. He writes about overcoming adversity and making our lives have meaning through personal efforts to do good and to be kind, no matter what happens. He notes that in order to move forward, we need to acknowledge the past, and if we are stuck, we need to get unstuck (p. 18). No matter what is in our way, his message is that we can get beyond it. What's more, we *need* to do it, for our own sake.

On the flip side, it is also helpful to acknowledge things that are *good* for you and that contribute to a sense of well-being and wholeness. When we acknowledge the gifts inherent in our lives, it fills us with joy. There are many aspects of our work as nurses that can make us feel heartful.

The environment in academia, as many will attest, is fraught with issues that can make the workplace unhealthy at times. Sometimes I really miss being with patients, but the students sustain me and my sense of purpose. Teaching end-of-life care, there are times when I am notably feeling compassion fatigued. You simply cannot help co-suffering, when teaching about dying, death, and bereavement. But I love what I do. I love teaching this topic and could not imagine doing anything else. It is the e-mails, notes, cards, and occasional visits from students who tell me what a difference my teachings have made for them that remind me when I seem to get overwhelmed and forget. The work I am doing *is* meaningful.

Think about the lives you have touched. You have no idea how far your reach has gone with your purposeful actions. One of my daughters told me today she bought an extra cup of coffee while in *Dunkin' Donuts* and "put it on the ledge." Just picturing that cup of coffee makes me smile. This act of kindness is thanks to students in a leadership class who, when I assigned an unguided teaching–learning creating change project, took it upon themselves to go around town to coffee shops to get store managers to institute the practice of "hanging coffee." Essentially, a customer goes into a coffee shop, and buys an extra cup of coffee. The store management then makes it known to the community (usually by posting signs) that extra cups of coffee are "hanging around" for those who cannot afford to buy one. This great idea came from a coffee shop in Prague called *The Hanging Coffee Café and Pub*. A student had gone to this café while visiting Prague and she shared the idea with her group members. They in turn shared the idea with their families, friends, and classmates, who shared the idea with others . . . it is at least 5 years later and here is my daughter, "hanging" cups of coffee. Random acts of kindness, paying it forward; these things are purposeful acts of caring that can make a huge difference.

If you think about it, nursing is a continual process of sometimes random, sometimes intentional, but always purposeful, acts of kindness. Our compassionate caring actions in nursing practice come at some of the most significant times of our patient's lives. What we do is so meaningful. Being mindfully aware and acknowledging the contributions we make in our day-to-day work nourishes and enhances our compassion contentment, leading us to feel ever more heartful.

Step 2: Recognition

The second step of *ART* is the Recognition that we always have choices, and then, with intention, we are able to choose those actions that will reaffirm our purpose. In this way, one may achieve a re-enchantment with one's life (and our life's purpose). Our lives are full of choices; they not only shape the path of each person's present and future, but also inform and transform the lives of others. And it is important to note that, "from a conventional viewpoint, we make 'bad choices.' But from a transcendental perspective, there are no wrong decisions only different lessons" (Millman, 2000, p. 138).

As Henry David Thoreau (1854/1995) noted, "We should be blessed if we lived in the present always, and took advantage of every accident that befell us" (p. 203). Things are happening in our day-to-day living that are very meaningful and could help us along our life journey, but many times we miss them entirely because we are not paying attention to our moments. I am referring to magical moments such as when a child smiles at you or when you walk out into a gloriously beautiful day and are met with melodious birdsong or a butterfly nectaring on a flower nearby (or perhaps flapping its wings!). However, I am also referring to what we may deem to be insignificant moments, events that we tend to shrug off as chance happenings, but which in actuality may be very important, if only we would recognize them as such.

Meaningful Coincidences

"Chance" happenings can be very meaningful, especially when we stop to reflect upon them. When something that is unlikely to happen does happen, and it is appreciably connected to some other thing, this is referred to as synchronicity or meaningful coincidence (Jung, 1973; Peat, 1987). I am a firm believer in synchronicity and have studied the phenomenon as it relates to grief healing (Todaro-Franceschi, 2006). Meaningful coincidences are purposeful changes—energy transformation—that emerge out of our wholeness; oneness (Todaro-Franceschi, 1998, 1999). People who pay attention (to the changes occurring) can be directed in momentous ways to actualize their potential; in other words, the synchronicity is transformative!

For years I had a *Celestine Prophecy* poster in my office to remind me to pay attention to my moments (Redfield, 1993). I no longer need the reminder to pay attention to the synchronicity occurring in my life, although I do not always follow up as I should. A case in point was when my husband and I traveled to Maui for our 25th wedding anniversary. While there, we hiked to one of only a few red beaches in the world, Kaihalulu (Roaring Sea) or Red Sand Beach. It was a difficult hike, very hilly and slippery, and parts of the trail had drastically eroded.

The trail wound through a very old cemetery, and many headstones had fallen below into the surf. It was very scenic and sad. As we rounded the last bend of this rugged trail, there was the most magnificent place—a bright red volcanic sand beach—contrasted against the turquoise blue ocean, with frothy white waves rolling into shore. I immediately noted that there were only six other people there; one was a man who had carried his child there on his back in an infant carrier. He had passed us along the trail, obviously much more comfortable with the rough terrain than we were. As we waded in the ocean, awestruck by this glorious place, a newlywed couple approached us and asked us to take a picture of them. We spoke with them briefly. Imagine our surprise to find that we lived less than a mile from each other, in Brooklyn, New York! I would have pursued the meaning of this synchronicity; however, it was their honeymoon, after all, and it seemed intrusive to prolong our goodbyes. Still, I often wonder why we met when we did, for how unlikely was it that we had? It really is a small world; when synchronicity occurs like this, we realize that it is all one.

Have you ever had a day where everything went smoothly and things you did not expect happened to make it all come together in a profoundly good way? Belitz and Lundstrom (1997) referred to these synchronicity events as "being in the flow:"

> In those times, we know we're in the right place at the right time doing the right thing. We feel both exhilarated and at peace, somehow connected to something larger and greater than ourselves. Life is rich with meaning, magic, and purpose. (p. xi)

When things *seem* to go wrong, I think perhaps it is synchronicity too. There are messages in everything, if only we take the time to recognize and reflect upon them. Realizing that things are connected can lead us to make choices we would never have thought of making.

We always have a choice in the matter!

Even when we think we do not have any choice in the matter, we always do. Doing nothing is a choice too! It is all one, and as such we are always participating, whether knowingly or unknowingly (Todaro-Franceschi, 1998, 1999). As nurse scholar and friend John Phillips always says, you cannot *not* participate! Recognition of choices can be enhanced by paying particular attention to what is going on in your moments and trying to keep track of them through such things as journaling or recording events and memories. Once you recognize the possible choices you have, then you can choose to take purposeful action to actualize some potentials rather than others. Always know that making a decision does not necessarily mean you cannot change your mind later. In fact, in most cases, you can easily change your mind and then make another choice. Of course, if you have carefully thought through your options and make a radical decision, it is unlikely you will want to go back and renege after the fact. What do I mean by radical decision? I mean a decision that results in a big change in your way of being in the world, and make no mistake, one that will transform other people's ways of being in the world too.

A Radical Decision

I worked for a time in a small community hospital first as per diem nursing staff and then as a full-time clinical supervisor of the intensive care unit and a medical surgical unit with some dedicated telemetry beds. Dedicated telemetry beds in this hospital meant that we had portable units, which were hooked up to patients, and strips were obtained on a regular basis. It did not mean that they were actually being monitored; in fact, most of the nursing staff who worked there had not been taught how to read rhythm strips and were only required to print out strips and place them in the patient's chart.

It was a rough place to work because the nurses were not well-respected by many of the physicians. It was one of those places that had what we call an "old boys club," a group of physicians who considered nurses to be handmaidens and little else. Even the top hospital administrator was one of those old boys. Naturally, staffing was a *big* problem. The hospital administration not only had a problem with bedside nurse retention, they also had difficulty keeping their nurse leaders. While I was working there, the director of nursing (DON) retired and the administration hired a new director. It immediately became apparent who buttered her bread. When she was not kissing up to her boss, she was "enforcing" rules and regulations.

One day, we had a code in the intensive care unit, and there was only one regular staff member along with two per diem nurses on duty. It was already a terrible day in that unit. There were seven patients and every one of them should have been one-to-one assignments. Having a code made it all the more horrific, putting both the patients and the staff at risk. Of course, I went up to the unit to assist the other nurses; there was no way I was staying out of there. Shortly after I arrived and was up to my neck multitasking, I was called to the phone because the DON wanted to speak with me. As I listened agape, she proceeded to tell me that I was to—right now!—go around the hospital and count the number of wheelchairs that did not have safety belts. I simply informed her that "now" was not a good time for me to leave the unit, that there was a code going on and they were short-staffed, and then I quickly hung up the phone. That woman actually called back to yell at me! I was pretty disturbed by her behavior; I waited until things calmed down on the unit and then did what she asked.

Not too long after, I had another experience, which left me reeling yet again. I was the weekend administrator on duty, meaning that all emergencies over the course of the weekend had to come to me. I received a call from one of our ED nurses who was concerned about a new admission; he told me he wanted to give me "a heads up" that there might be a problem. The nurse proceeded to tell me that the patient came in with chest pain. He believed that the patient was experiencing a myocardial infarction (MI) and, although he had told the physician this, the physician on duty had insisted the patient be admitted to the telemetry unit. To this I responded, "We cannot do that"—but in fact, it had already been done. I immediately went to the telemetry unit and found this patient alone in a private room, with a portable telemetry monitor at his side. What good was that, I thought? One look at the patient told me that the ED nurse was correct and that we needed to quickly get this patient up to the ICU where he could be properly monitored and cared for.

I was upset with the physician who knew it was our hospital policy that all patients being ruled out for MI were to be directly admitted to the ICU. I notified him via phone that the patient would have to be moved. His response was to scream into the phone that I was "just a nurse" and that I had no right whatsoever to question him, or to make any decisions regarding patient admissions. I had no choice but to call the chief of cardiology, who lived nearby. Before I could blink my eyes, it seemed, the chief had arrived to assess the patient. Of course, the patient had to be sent to the ICU and that meant the physician on call, who was already so irate, had to transfer one of the patients out of the ICU to make room for this new patient.

Later on in the day, when I was making rounds, I was confronted by the physician who asked me to step into the lounge area to speak privately. He proceeded to literally scream at me and swung his hands in my face. I was perceptibly shaken but determined to hold my ground. So I told him he had no right to speak to me like that and I walked away. I wrote up the incident and submitted it to our DON the following Monday.

Never hearing anything further about it from the DON, I assumed that it was being taken care of and that the physician would at least be reprimanded for his inappropriate behavior. Imagine my dismay and anger when I heard from one of the other clinical supervisors that the director was investigating the way I related to physicians, by asking the MDs whether my responses to them "were appropriate!" I went to a few of the nurses and physicians to confirm that this was indeed occurring and left work at the end of the day fuming. I sat down that evening, acknowledged that there was a problem, and made a list of my possible choices:

- I could go to work and act like nothing had happened (yeah, right).
- I could go to work and ask the director why she would choose to investigate one of her staff rather than support and advocate for her (and nothing would happen).
- I could take it over her head to the hospital administrator, who was an MD and had been in the position for years (and nothing would happen).
- I could quit the position.

So, what did I do? You guessed it; I quit. I am proud to say that I did it with real flare. I wrote my resignation, to be effective at 3 p.m. the next day. In it, I shared my concerns for a hospital administration that did not put the best interests of the patients first and foremost. Of course, I also shared my concerns for a workplace that did not sufficiently support its nursing staff and leaders.

The next morning I went in at 8 a.m., left the resignation letter for the director, who was not yet in her office, cleaned and packed up my office, and then made my rounds. While I did so, I informed everyone I would be out of there at the end of the day. I then spent the remainder of the day saying "hell no!" to physicians and staff alike who stopped by my office to beg me to reconsider.

To leave that place the way I did was a radical decision and one I have never regretted, although I did lose my sick time and a few weeks of vacation pay because I did not give the mandatory 2-week notice. Some folks thought I cut my nose off to spite my face; I thought it was well worth it. I am a firm believer in the "take this job and shove it" mentality, when the job is putting you at risk. That job was putting me at risk for a lot

of ugliness. Had I stayed, the ugly head of burnout would surely have surfaced eventually—and when I think about it, of all the possible ugly issues
that could have surfaced, that might have been the prettiest of the bunch.
Making another list of the possible changes, depending upon making
different choices, is helpful too. In this case, here are a few possibilities,
had I chosen to stay there:

- Having units with inadequate staff could result in serious errors or
  omissions, causing more harm than good to the patients and as the
  covering supervisor I could be jeopardizing my RN license (e.g., if
  something were to happen to the patient as a result of his being
  admitted to the wrong unit, I could be charged with negligence).

- Emotional, physical, and spiritual exhaustion (compassion fatigue
  and/or burnout) can lead to altered health status and serious,
  perhaps even life-threatening, illness.

At the end of the day, the job was not worth it!

If you are having difficulty recognizing the choices you have and you
have no one to be a sounding board, you can try pulling up a chair and
having a chat with yourself. In fact, even if you have others to talk with,
occasionally it is helpful to just talk to yourself. Indeed, I do it often and
consider it a sign of normalcy. Eric Maisel (2005), famed creativity coach,
suggests pulling up two chairs and alternating your position, first being
yourself and then being your coach. When you sit in the first chair you
can be you, and when you sit in the second chair you become your own
coach. In this way you can coach yourself to make choices that will lead
you toward a plan of action to reaffirm your purpose in nursing.

Step 3: Turning Outward Toward Self and Other

The third step, like the others, is meant to be ongoing and entails a Turning
outward toward self and others. It is when one becomes aware that through
reconnection, not only with self but also with others (our loved ones, coworkers, and patients), we can remain content in our work and feel heartful. If we are compassion fatigued, reconnecting with ourselves and others
can help us to heal (the reconnect contention!).

Nurses are human beings taking care of human beings. We need to frequently remind ourselves of this as we go about our day-to-day work.
Reiterating my earlier words, we are *not* robots. When discussing how to
keep compassion fatigue at bay through the reconnect contention, I accent-
uate making time to see things you normally would not notice. We can use
this practice in both our personal and professional lives. At the end of a work
day, how often do we go home at night and barely notice our loved ones?
The dog's tail is wagging as you walk through the door and you tell him to

get out of your way. Your husband, wife, or children are trying to tell you things and you are completely zoning them out. Does this sound familiar?

In our work environment, oftentimes we lose sight of the person in the bed, so intent are we to do all the multitasking that needs to be done. Nurse Doris Hines (1992) noted that we should "enfold the skills and technologies within the relationship rather than performing the task according to safety requirements and as the main function of the time spent together" (p. 303). I regularly ask my fellow nurses, "What if, when we are with a patient, taking care of IVs, Foleys, and wounds, we make the focus the *patient*, rather than the things associated with the person? What if we encourage our patients to talk to us as we take care of the mundane day-to-day activities of nursing, the things we barely think about as we are doing them because they have become second nature to us?"

It is important to take time to *see* our patients, really see them. How often do we notice the color of a patient's hair or eyes? These are small things, perhaps, but nevertheless a beginning step in reconnecting with others. Our purpose as professional carers is to provide care, to heal, and we cannot do that effectively without forming some *connection* with those we care for every day. To remain disconnected only feeds the illusion that all things are separate. It is unrewarding to feel this way and over time can only generate a growing discontent with work and life in general.

It may be a human defense mechanism to distance oneself from painful experiences; however, to keep loving what we do in nursing, we need to remind ourselves time and again that we are *allowed to feel*; essentially, we need to get closer to others rather than put more distance between us. We need to *Turn outward*, toward ourselves and others, even when doing so means that we feel *more*, not less.

Nussbaum (1996) pointed out that:

> Equipped with her general conception of human flourishing, the spectator looks at a world in which people suffer hunger, disability, disease, slavery, through no fault of their own or beyond their fault. In her pity she acknowledges that goods such as food, health, citizenship, freedom, do all matter. Yet she acknowledges, as well, that it is uncertain whether she herself will remain among the safe and privileged ones to whom such goods are stably guaranteed. She acknowledges that the lot of the poor might be (or become) hers. This leads her to *turn her thoughts outward* [Italics mine], from her own current comfortable situation to the structure of society's allocation of goods and resources. For, given the uncertainty of life, she will be inclined to want a society in which the lot of the worst off—of the poor, of people defeated in war, of women, of servants—is as good as it can be. (p. 36)

Through our empathetic concern, we recognize that "I" is "we"—it is all one. Mindfully remaining aware of our "we-ness" can keep us loving what we do.

Healing our workforce must entail a reawakening of what Capra and Steindl-Rast (1991) referred to as a sense of belonging to the universe. Studies on how spiritual experiences and practices can lead to a transformation of consciousness suggest that "altruism and compassion may arise as natural consequences of experiences of interconnectedness and oneness" and that these transformational experiences "appear to lead to shifts in perspective and changes in one's sense of self and self in relationship to others" (Vieten, Amorok, & Schlitz, 2006, p. 915).

By encouraging experiences of connectedness and oneness, we may enhance our altruistic compassionate nature, which is integral to the nurse's authentic self. We do not have to accept compassion fatigue and/or burnout as the costs of caring; with intention, we can make choices that help us to reaffirm our purpose and actively sidestep feeling dissatisfied and disenchanted with our work.

Eckhart Tolle (2005) wrote that all of us have both an inner purpose and an outer purpose. Our inner purpose is for each of us to awaken; it is a collective purpose for all human beings: "Your inner purpose is an essential part of the purpose of the whole, the universe and its emerging intelligence" (p. 258). To awaken means to become aware of the connectedness-oneness. It means to be able to rid oneself of the ego or what he refers to as the "illusory self" (p. 27), along with the corresponding idea that we are separate from everything else. With true awakening, we can perceive the patterns of the whole and the words "I," "me," "my," and so forth, disappear, and in their stead it is "we" and "us." On the other hand, each of us has an outer purpose that is unique—it varies from one person to another and it is fluid—it changes over time.

When both our inner purpose and outer purpose are in alignment, we are in a state of "awakened doing," which essentially means our acts are more closely in tune with the purposeful actions of the universe (Tolle, p. 294). Tolle (2005) suggests that we can purposefully do "awakened doing" through the use of three modalities: (1) acceptance, (2) joy, and (3) enthusiasm (p. 295). Each of these modalities is appropriate at different times and all of them can help us tap into what he calls "the creative power of the universe" (p. 295).

APPLYING *ART* FOR COMPASSION CONTENTMENT

Having considered the positive aspect of professional quality of life—compassion contentment—in previous chapters, we can take *ART* and apply it to hold and enhance a sense of heartfulness. When you use *ART* to enhance compassion contentment you are, in essence, doing an appreciative inquiry or self-interview. Appreciative inquiry is a means to mindfully identify the positive aspects of our lives so that as we move through life we can repeatedly experience and appreciate what brings us joy and happiness (also see Chapter 11).

Try the following:

- *Acknowledge* a good feeling from an experience you had at work, something that made you feel glad to be a nurse. What did you choose to do that day that made it all seem worthwhile and that had you leaving at the end of the day feeling content about your day's work? Did you look forward to going to work the following day? Acknowledge how good you felt while you were in a specific moment. What were you doing and how did you feel while doing it? Jot down the things that contributed to your good feeling.

- *Recognize* that one always has choices and then choose appropriate actions to reaffirm purpose. Going back to that good day at work, can you identify the choices you made that contributed to the day turning out the way it did? Is having a good moment or day an anomaly in your work life? If so, why? What are the obstacles? What can you *do* to make it a regular happening? What did you choose to do that day that made it all seem worthwhile? Can you make the same or similar choices today? If not, why not? If so, what is preventing you right now, this moment, from doing it?

- *Turn* outward toward yourself and others. Can you take the positive experience you had and reproduce it? Were you able to connect with your patients, loved ones, and coworkers? Grasp your sense of well-being from that time. Reconnect with those feelings.

Hopefully, as you read and work on each of these steps, they will encourage you to be present with *yourself* and to be aware of your connection to others. *Combined **ART** can be thought of as awakening.*

TURNING POINTS EXERCISE: LOOKING BACKWARD TO LOOK FORWARD

When applying *ART*, you focus on awareness of turning points, connection to others (and the environment), and one's place (individually and collectively) in the unfolding present.

Find a quiet place, a pen and paper, and about 15 minutes of "me" time. Sit and reflect upon your career. Did my story of applying for a job at Macy's resonate with you? Has there been a time when you seriously considered leaving nursing? What about right now? When you first entered the profession of nursing, what goals did you have? What did you think you would be doing? Are you doing it? Have you met your goals? Have your goals changed? Make a list here.

Goals	Met	Not Met
1. _____	____	____
2. _____	____	____
3. _____	____	____
4. _____	____	____

The goal is to get clarity about what your priorities are and then act on them. While many of us feel we have no choice, remember, we always do (yes, I am trying hard to brainwash you!). It is a matter of being able to recognize what choices we have and which ones are more important for each of us at particular points in time. What are your priorities? Through mindful awareness of what is going on right now, in this moment, you can discover your options and act accordingly. If you have not met the goals that you previously set for yourself, you will need to explore the reason(s) why. The following chapters will help you to get further clarity.

KEY POINTS

- *ART* is a healing model comprised of three steps designed to help address professional quality-of-life issues: (1) *A*cknowledgement of a feeling or problem; (2) *R*ecognition of the possible choices one has and then choosing which actions to take to reaffirm purpose in one's work life and, (3) *T*urning outward toward self and other. This is done by making a conscious effort to reconnect with oneself and others (AKA, the "reconnect contention").
- *ART* is ongoing and steps may overlap. The key is to be mindfully aware of our moments and actions.
- With intention we can find meaning in our work and be heartful (at least most of the time!)

Part 3

THE BAD AND THE UGLY: COMPASSION FATIGUE AND BURNOUT

There can be no transforming of darkness into light and of apathy into movement without emotion.
—Carl G. Jung

Chapter 6

A HEAVY HEART HURTS

*Heavy hearts, like heavy clouds in the sky, are best
relieved by the letting of a little water.*
—ANTOINE RIVAROL

KEY TOPICS

- Compassion fatigue
- Primary and secondary trauma
- Incivility in the workplace
- Substance abuse

The very same qualities that make us excel as carers also put us at risk for compassion fatigue. Fundamentally, being compassionate and feeling compelled to care sets us up to be hurt.

While I was writing this book, I attended a conference sponsored by the National Institute of Nursing Research, where a number of brilliant people gathered together to explore where we have been and where we are going with palliative and end-of-life care. The title of the conference, coincidentally, was, "The Science of Compassion." The kickoff for this summit was a town hall discussion on ethical issues in end-of-life care. The topic turned to the vulnerability of people who are dying; however, it became glaringly apparent during the discussion that in designating some people as more or less vulnerable, we might be doing a disservice to some or all. Who is it that decides who is vulnerable and who is not? The bottom line is that all people are vulnerable at different points in their lives, and that, of course, includes us nurses. Our recognition of human vulnerability is in large part the basis of compassionate caring and is also the source of compassion fatigue.

DEFINING COMPASSION FATIGUE

Compassion fatigue is a syndrome that carers may develop when they internalize pain or anguish related to other people in their work environment. As noted earlier, the term *compassion fatigue* is ambiguous and is often used interchangeably with secondary traumatic stress (STS) and, on occasion, vicarious trauma.[1] It is sometimes referred to as a lesser (or unique form) of burnout.

Some of the most inclusive work on the subject has been written by trauma study pioneer Charles Figley (1995, 2002a, 2002b), who thinks that compassion fatigue is a more user-friendly term than STS, which is closely aligned with post-traumatic stress disorder (PTSD).[2] He believes that the modern-day description of this syndrome is equivalent to his early depiction of secondary victimization as well as the similar concept of "emotional contagion."[3] Basically, when carers become preoccupied with another's experience (of being traumatized), we too are traumatized (Figley, 1995, 2002b).

Figley (2002a) also described compassion fatigue as a chronic lack of self-care, and this definition is in keeping with Joinson's (1992) portrayal of compassion fatigue. It has been said that the most basic thing nurses provide in the delivery of care to others is ourselves, and unless we can find ways to continuously renew ourselves from the drain associated with our nursing practice, we will not only lose energy but also enthusiasm for our work (Joinson, 1992). What is always implicit in any description of the syndrome is that those who develop compassion fatigue are, on some level, internalizing pain and suffering from their relationship with others in the workplace, usually co-suffering with another human being, and it is manifesting itself in harmful ways on a multidimensional level. If it is not recognized and tended to, it can spiral out of control and may eventually result in burnout (Benson & Magraith, 2005; Figley, 2002b).

Who Is at Risk?

Nurses who work in areas where patients usually do not return to a previous level of wellness are especially at risk of compassion fatigue; however, it is important to realize that we bear witness to suffering in all areas of health care. Palliative care nurse pioneers Betty Ferrell and Nessa Coyle (2008) emphasized this in a book on the nature of suffering and the goals of nursing. Suffering is part of the human condition, and while we each may be able to describe some universal idea of what it means to suffer, the lived experience of suffering is unique for every person. Consequently, none of us can ever assume that suffering is or is not taking place; we need to look deeper than the surface.

People with chronic, and what are referred to as life-limiting illnesses, as well as acute, life-threatening illnesses, are often treated aggressively, and treatments can result in additional suffering for them and their loved ones. Their suffering is a part of the nurse's daily work, and whether or not the nurse acknowledges it, he or she internalizes at least some of the anguish. Even a seemingly benign task such as obtaining bed scale weights might be quite traumatic for both the cared for and the carer. And, while I may still shudder to recall those bed scale weight days in the ICU (and really I do!), other coworkers may not; such is the uniqueness of human beings.

Since what is traumatic to one person may not be to another, it is imperative to recognize the possibility that someone might be traumatized, even when we think not. It is also important to explore what the term *trauma* implies to you. You may realize that some of the experiences you have had were very traumatic, although at the time you did not realize it (see also Chapter 10).

BUTTERFLY POWER: SUBTLE INFLUENCES AND BEING TRAUMATIZED

Traumatic stressors are described as those things that might contribute to the development of the syndromes of compassion fatigue and burnout, and they can be primary or secondary in nature (Stamm, 2002, 2010). Primary trauma can be anything that directly affects us. In the workplace, experiences such as getting hit on the job or being browbeaten (mentally abused) or bullied by colleagues and/or management count as primary trauma, whereas witnessing the suffering of others is considered secondary trauma.

Repeated or prolonged exposure to trauma, which is relational in nature, can lead to the sudden occurrence of compassion fatigue. This is similar to that night I broke down in tears and could not take one more night of caring for John, or that WHAM! I experienced years ago, when I woke up one day and realized I no longer looked forward to going to work.

Not too long ago, while speaking with some nurse colleagues, I was surprised to find out that a few of them did not consider working with people who are in the ICU to be a source of trauma. This goes back to the point about our unique perceptions of who may or may not be vulnerable and what may or may not be traumatic. It is also indicative of the continuing lack of knowledge related to the syndromes of compassion fatigue and burnout. Not being able to recognize and understand what might contribute to these syndromes puts everyone at a disadvantage.

It has been noted that, "All of us who attempt to heal the wounds of others will ourselves be wounded; it is, after all, inherent in the relationship" (Hilfiker, 1985, p. 207). How is it that some nurses might not think that working with ill people is at all traumatizing? Perhaps it is for the very same reason that many of us in health care continue to use terms like "passed away" or "expired" instead of "dead" or "died." Technologizing or dehumanizing suffering makes it commonplace and distant rather than up front and center. After all, it is our job to provide care *no matter what*, to get all the medications in, to chart everything, to change the dressings, and so forth; never mind that we are walking in and out of rooms full of people who are scared and deathly ill.

There are a lot of things in the profession of nursing that can contribute to the development of compassion fatigue. Some of the contributors may be overt, while others are more covert or subtle—basically, anything that results in one's *heart feeling heavy*.

Briggs and Peat (1999), in their discussion on "butterfly power," describe how small subtle changes can transform things on a large scale. In relation to compassion fatigue and burnout, it is the *negative* subtle influences that occur in many systems that are a cause for concern.[4] They note that people may consciously conform to the traditional or expected workings within a system and automatically go along with the norm in order to survive. This kind of process is comprised of a negative feedback loop—the same behavior pattern is exhibited over and over again. Unfortunately, the health care system has many such negative subtle influences and some not-so-subtle influences too. Take, for instance, the story of a nurse who was at the top of her class upon graduation. She was hired to work on an oncology unit in a major teaching hospital renowned for excellent care. Having taken a course on death, dying, and bereavement, she felt she had something to offer this particular population of patients and was extremely happy with her first position working as a nurse. The following was shared with me shortly after she began to work on the unit:

> *Reality has officially set in and it bothers me so much. I want to sit with my patients, hold their hands, cry with them, and provide them with true presence but my preceptor is always rushing me out of the room saying I have too many things to do. I know she is right, but I feel so awful at times. I am fortunate in that every single patient thus far has opened up to me in so many ways, and many have cried to me, telling me things that they have not told other nurses on the unit. I feel so honored to have their trust and feel that I am violating my relationship with them because of my workload. My unit is one step below an ICU and I have six patients minimum every shift. I try hard but find myself going home sad many nights. It got to the point where I was waking up the last couple of weeks and telling myself how much I dislike that unit, and your words came into my mind: "When you wake up feeling like you hate your job, it's time to go."*

*The nurses on this unit are extremely competent but I have seen com-
passion displayed by only two other nurses, who are both coincidentally leaving next week. I have stayed there because I know that I am
making a difference, no matter how small, and I see the look in many
of my patients' eyes when I go in to say good-bye to them at the end of
my shift and when they ask me if I will come back the following day to
be their nurse.*

*I'm trying the techniques that you taught me, such as talking to them
as I give them their medications, holding their hands as I take their
pulse; I cover them when they seem cold; I lower myself at eye-to-
eye level to let them know I am truly listening, and I thank you
so much for teaching me those skills in our class on death and
dying . . . . I have spoken of you many times on my unit. I have even
considered suggesting that you be brought in to show these nurses
the things that you showed us, because most of the nurses are burnt
out and provide no compassion whatsoever.*

*I love nursing, so please do not misunderstand my comments. I just
need to find my own style of providing the care that my patients
require without losing the three essential components that are important in nursing: compassion, caring, and commitment to my patients.*

Each time a nurse shares a story such as this, I want to cry for all of us.
How is it possible that some nurses have allowed themselves to harden
so much?

Obviously, the harried environment of this unit did not support the
new nurse's conception of what it meant to provide quality care to her
patients. Despite this, she managed to withstand the negative subtle influences of her work environment and eventually made a choice to move to
another place of employment rather than join in on the negative feedback
loop to become one of the automated, seemingly uncaring nurses on that
particular unit.

Both primary and secondary traumas are exemplified in this new
nurse's situation. Secondary trauma is evidenced by her identifying with
the suffering of her patients; however, she felt gifted to bear witness to
that suffering. She knew that by doing so, she was doing something
good for her patients and also herself. This is a buffer, really, for her
acknowledgement of the contribution she was making helped to sustain
her sense of purpose. At the same time, the unit pace and the other
nurses working with her were not supportive and did not value her conception of what it meant to be a "good nurse."

Primary trauma arose from her frequently being the butt of negative
commentary, such as being told she was too slow and not cut out for
this work. She regularly overheard the staff talking about her, saying

unpleasant and, on occasion, even racist things. This distressed her even more; unfortunately, her story is *not* an oddity in nursing.

Joinson (1992) described how compassion fatigue can emerge in relation to how we are providing care for others, but she also noted that our coworkers can contribute to its development. She wrote, "When the people around you are tense, impatient, and hurried, you may be swept into the same reactions. Nurses who are tired, indifferent or cynical, can sap your own energy and enthusiasm" (p. 118). Notably, Joinson was alluding to the precursor for what we refer to in current day as bullying or incivility in the workplace; it is the indifferent and/or cynical nurse who treats coworkers, and on occasion, patients and their loved ones, with a lack of respect. Some, if not the majority, of these bullying nurses are probably themselves suffering from burnout.

Incivility in the Workplace

When you are in a new job as a new nurse, with a significant learning curve to enable you to go from the ideal to the real, it is unconscionable to think that senior nurses would be cruel and uncaring. Yet, the literature shows that nurses frequently do not treat their coworkers nicely. What is more, far too often, students and *new* nurses are the targeted victims of bullying in the workplace (McKenna, Smith, Poole, & Coverdale, 2003; Thomas & Burk, 2009). In the previous exemplar, the subtle and not-so-subtle negative influences that were portrayed by the behavior of the nurses on the unit can also be explored from the position of those nurses themselves. Some of the questions to ponder include asking why they were criticizing, insulting, and devaluing the nurse for her meticulous attention to her patients. What made them that way? Is their behavior a means of distancing themselves from their own unhappiness? I cannot imagine that, at the end of the day, nurses who are cruel to others are happy people.

Incivility or bullying in the workplace can be both a symptom of compassion fatigue and burnout and also a contributing factor in the development of compassion fatigue and burnout. It plays a large part in work dissatisfaction overall and can be devastating for the recipients, with physical, psychological, and spiritual ramifications. What has been given little attention is the fact that it is also devastating for the perpetrators, because in a very real sense these nurses have completely lost their sense of purpose as carers. The pendulum has swung completely the other way.

There are two types of workplace bullying: (a) horizontal or lateral violence (also known as peer-to-peer aggression, because the bully and the bullied are equal in stature or employment level), and (b) hierarchical or vertical violence (where the bully is superordinate, for example, a head nurse or supervisor) (Broome & Williams-Evans, 2011; Longo, 2007; Thomas & Burk, 2009). Unfortunately, it seems that most bullies in the workplace are in management, where by virtue of their positions of power, they are able to control the victims (Cleary, Hunt, & Horsfall, 2010). Both types of bullying behavior foster a hostile working environment. In cases where nurses observe a coworker being repeatedly bullied, although they themselves are not the recipients, they too suffer from bearing witness. And because of the antagonistic environment, the witnesses of bullying behavior may join in and take part, even if they do not want to do so—they might go along to get along—and what is known as "mobbing" can occur. As a result, the bullied (suffering from primary trauma) and the witnesses to the bullying (co-suffering—secondary trauma) are at increased risk of compassion fatigue, which ultimately results in a collective wound.

Victims of bullying have been found to manifest various patterns of mental and/or physical distress, and, in fact, several studies have shown a distinct similarity between the symptoms arising from bullying and PTSD (Bilgel, Aytac, & Bayram, 2006; Ramos, 2006; see Chapter 10 for a further discussion of PTSD). Recipients of bullying may manifest anxiety, depression, low self-esteem, eating disorders, weight loss, high blood pressure, and angina, among many other things (Broome & Williams-Evans, 2011).

Toxic work environments where bullying regularly takes place leads to nurse absenteeism and poor staff retention, which then result in financial losses for the institution. Poor work relationships impact not only staff satisfaction but also performance, contributing to emotional exhaustion, the purportedly cardinal manifestation of burnout (Cleveland Clinic, 2011). Ultimately, the care rendered to those who are in need of our caring is negatively affected and, thus, attaining and maintaining a culture of safety for *both* the cared for and the carers become impossible:

> Intimidating and disruptive behaviors can foster medical errors, contribute to poor patient satisfaction and preventable adverse outcomes, increase the cost of care, and cause qualified clinicians and managers to seek new positions in more professional environments. (Governance Institute, 2009, p. 22)

As incivility in health care work environments has become an increasing concern, the Joint Commission (2008) and the Center for American Nurses (2008) have been quick to advocate for the abolishment of bullying in the workplace, and strategies have been identified such as the development of codes of acceptable behavior in organizations, increased education, and zero-tolerance policies. To some extent, all these may work; however, it is crucial that we try to understand what is behind the acts of incivility. I see it as another glaring indication of a wounded workforce. Without an understanding and focus on the removal of potential causes, I doubt that we can eradicate it from the workplace.

Death Overload

Where nurses work can contribute to the development of compassion fatigue. In areas where there is a higher incidence of dying and death, suffering is more visible, and, thus, larger numbers of nurses are at risk. *Death overload*, a term used to denote having experienced the death of too many patients in a short period or having worked with a patient for too long a time prior to the person dying, is also a form of traumatic stress (Vachon, 1993). Critical care, trauma, and emergency department nurses and those working in oncology and palliative care are more apt to experience death overload. My firsthand experiences working in many of these areas and my years of teaching nurses prompt me to say, with some conviction, that the most troubling thing for a great number of nurses who work in these areas is to *face death* (and the suffering that often accompanies it). By this I mean not only us having to face the patient but also the family members of those patients who are dying (see Chapter 9).

There is some evidence to show that many individuals who provide care that they believe to be medically futile (care that will not lead to eventual cure or a better quality of life) develop compassion fatigue and burnout. For instance, Meltzer and Huckabay (2004) studied 60 critical care nurses' perceptions of futile care and its effect on the development of burnout. They found a positive correlation between the critical care nurses' emotional exhaustion scores and morally distressful situations where the care provided was considered to be medically futile. I return to this topic in further depth in Chapter 9.

MANIFESTATIONS OF COMPASSION FATIGUE

Signs and symptoms of compassion fatigue are abundant and highly individualized, but for the most part, they usually go unnoticed by those who are experiencing the phenomenon (see Exhibit 6.1). Because compassion fatigue is also considered to arise from co-suffering, we would do well to recall the manifestations of suffering, noting that it is existential and encompasses the entire being. A common response *to* suffering *is* suffering.

EXHIBIT 6.1: SOME TYPICAL SIGNS OF COMPASSION FATIGUE (AND BURNOUT)

Behavior Changes

Inability to maintain balance of empathy and objectivity
Depression

(Continued)

EXHIBIT 6.1: SOME TYPICAL SIGNS OF COMPASSION FATIGUE
(AND BURNOUT) (*Continued*)

Anger
Blaming
Irritability
Chronic lateness
Overworking
Exaggerated startle response
Difficulty focusing or concentrating
Substance abuse
Eating disturbances
Disrupted sleep patterns
Avoiding or dreading work
Calling out sick more often

Feelings

Heart heavy compassion fatique
Diminished sense of personal accomplishment
Decreased sense of purpose
Less able to feel joy or happiness
Low self-esteem
High self-expectations
Helplessness and hopelessness
Numbness
Empty hearted (burnout)
Disinterested and detached
Disillusioned
Apathy

Physical Changes

Chronic fatigue
Exhaustion (physical, emotional, or both)
Frequent headaches
Gastrointestinal complaints
Hypertension
Cardiac symptoms such as chest pain or tachycardia
Sleep disturbances
Muscle tension, aches, and pains
Frequent or lingering illness
Difficulty focusing
Anxiety

We have no real way of knowing how our own health is transformed by the occurrence of compassion fatigue, for as nurse Brenda Sabo (2006) noted, there has been little focus on how our nursing work may be changing our health status. In fact, all the seminal research that has been done on health status using nurses as participants could not possibly have taken this piece of the *whole* into consideration, making those research findings a bit skewed. Going back to that new nurse: She has type I diabetes. During her time on that unit, she suffered frequent episodes of severe hypoglycemia along with loss of appetite and difficulty sleeping, in addition to the terrible emotional upheaval she experienced. Her life was literally being threatened by her work. So in answer to the question, "Can we accurately capture the consequences of caring work?" (Sabo, 2006, p. 136), it becomes clear that we cannot. The whole is far too complex and each case is highly individualized.

The list in Exhibit 6.1 is not meant to be all-inclusive. Realize too that not all of the signs and symptoms have to be evident for one to be suffering from compassion fatigue and there is also significant overlap with the symptoms of burnout. I touch upon a few of the signs of compassion fatigue in greater depth here; others have been or are discussed in other places. Again, I am really trying to emphasize the *whole*.

Turning Away

In nursing and in other health care professions, there is a high incidence of substance abuse. It is estimated that the incidence of substance abuse in nursing mirrors the rates of national levels of 10% to 12% of the population (Clark & Farnsworth, 2006), although some research suggests that it might be a bit lower or higher (Ramer, 2008). In one study, oncology nurses were found to have a higher incidence of substance abuse than other specialty groups (Trinkoff & Storr, 1998), which, when looked at from the perspective of compassion fatigue, does seem to make sense. Patients with cancer often suffer from both the disease and the treatments. Nurses who work in oncology are frequently providing care while wondering why the treatments are being continued; or they may be stopping care while wondering why it is not being continued. There is a lot to "co-suffer with" in oncology.

Substance abuse and eating disturbances, when they occur in relation to some experience or event, are considered a form of self-medicating. I consider them an indication of how people turn *away from*, rather than turn *toward*, something. The something we need to turn toward is ourselves; we need to reconnect with or confront whatever is bothering us before the destructive behaviors harm us. We need to go to the places that scare us. This is easier said than done. Indeed, it can be very difficult to recognize that there is a problem and to face it head on.

A general rule of thumb is, if you are drinking or taking medication as a way to relax or de-stress on a regular basis, or if you turn to food, you are self-medicating and abusing the drug or overindulging in food. If you find that you cannot go without a drink or a drug, then there is a possibility that you are psychologically, if not physically, already dependent on it. If your loved ones have voiced concern over your drinking or drug habits, that is also a clue that you need to evaluate your behavior.

I once worked on a unit where quite a few of the staff were abusing alcohol; back then I did not realize it, but looking back I can see where, if things had not changed, I might have developed a problem myself. Many of the folks who were on the night shift would stop on the way home for wine coolers and/or beer. I recall that, on occasion, when I got home from a particularly difficult night I would go and sit in the garden drinking a wine cooler at 9 in the morning to unwind because I could not sleep. Did I know it was a step *away* from what I needed to be doing for myself? No. I was probably very fortunate that we had to relocate while I was still working at that particular place. I am not sure I would have been able to recognize that there was a problem endemic to the unit I was working on at the time. Today, I do recognize it. I am hoping that some of you, while reading this, have an AHA! moment too.

One of the biggest problems with individuals who are abusing drugs or alcohol is that they do not recognize they have a problem before it gets out of control. If you are leaning on a bottle (of alcohol or pills or some other form of drug), or maybe you are leaning on too many Twinkies, you have choices that you can make to work on healing. You can choose to speak with your health care provider about it and/or also seek help from your employee assistance program (EAP). You need not worry about confidentiality; you are protected and there is no stigma associated with seeking help for addictive behaviors. Nurses are people too (although it might not seem like this is so, it is a mandate that all employers have an EAP). Today employers realize that it is far more cost effective to help impaired nurses rehabilitate rather than lose them entirely.

A related issue in health care workplaces that has not been given much attention is the associated trauma to nurses who are working with those who they know to be substance abusers. They may become morally distressed because, on the one hand, these nurses are compelled to report their concerns, knowing that it is a matter of legal and ethical obligation to do so. At the same time, they co-suffer with their coworker, and can easily become compassion fatigued.

In bearing witness to or discovering drug diversion by a coworker, nurses often feel anger, betrayal, and grief (Ramer, 2008). It is important for them to seek assistance themselves—to turn outward and acknowledge the problem rather than turn away from it. Needless to say, the way nurse leaders support, or conversely, do not support, the nurses on units where drug diversion has been discovered can make or break the sense of communality among staff, which in turn affects overall retention and productivity. If not adequately supported, collective wounds will fester and the environment can become toxic, but with compassionate leadership, healing will occur (see also Chapter 11).

If you are abusing substances and become addicted, or know of a nurse who is, supportive programs such as Alcoholics Anonymous, Narcotics Anonymous, and Overeaters Anonymous are tried-and-true programs with much success. In most states, there are now programs for impaired nurses, which may be called peer assistance or diversion programs. In all cases, nurses are assisted in regaining their former lives. (Please see the resource section for further information.)

CAN COMPASSION FATIGUE BE EVADED?

In earlier chapters I stressed the importance of compassion—as both a virtue and excellence in nursing. Here and there I have emphasized that we do not have to accept compassion fatigue as a consequence of caring work. We can take steps to alleviate it and also sometimes prevent it. For each of us it is a matter of finding the appropriate balance.

Perry (2008) highlighted reasons why exemplary oncology nurses seem to avoid compassion fatigue (p. 87). In one study she identified seven nurses whose practice was considered exemplary by their coworkers. Four of the nurses worked on a palliative care unit; the others worked in hospice or oncology. She engaged in conversations with each of the participants on the subject of compassion fatigue, after which she analyzed the transcripts for shared themes.

The seven nurses shared three main characteristics in their practice, which I noted in an earlier chapter: moments of connection, making moments matter, and energizing moments (Perry, 2008). All of these themes resonate with ideas of peak experiences, flow, second wind, and, in general, self-actualization. All are contingent on our ability to connect with self and other and on our ability to compassionately care. When we remain true to our authentic caring nature as we go about our practice— when we keep first and foremost in our hearts and minds the meaning and purpose of our work—it can help us to recognize and heal from, as well as avert, compassion fatigue.

APPLYING *ART* FOR COMPASSION FATIGUE

If you are suffering from compassion fatigue, being mindfully aware of your actions as you go about doing things in your day-to day activities can help to heal your wounds. Does any of the preceding resonate with you? Having picked up this book, it is likely that you do recognize there is a problem somewhere, so the hardest step has been taken already; now it is a matter of making choices that turn you back on the path to happiness and well-being. You are already applying *ART* here!

Step 1: Acknowledge Feelings (or a Wound That Needs Healing)

Bearing witness to one's own feelings, especially suffering, is difficult but necessary in order to enhance professional quality of life and heal from compassion fatigue. How do you feel when you are going into work? Are you looking forward to work or are you dreading it? Do you feel tired? Review the signs and symptoms in Exhibit 6.1. Complete the secondary traumatic stress/compassion fatigue part of Stamm's (2010) ProQOL tool in the appendix at the end of the book (Appendix A). Remember, all of this is meant as a guide to help you become more aware of your situation and whether there is a problem. It is not meant to be diagnostic but rather is a contemplative exercise.

Look *toward yourself* as you go about your day. Note how you act with others and how you react to others. Pay attention to what might be irritating or upsetting you over the course of your work day. Reflect on your moments while you are living them. Jot things down as you become aware of them.

If you have identified that you are compassion fatigued, you need to explore possible turning points and try to establish what factors in your work may have contributed to it. Looking back, can you recognize when you began to feel the way you are feeling? Depending on your circumstances, there may be more than one thing that you need to address. Once you are aware of the contributing factors, you can begin the second step.

Step 2: Recognize Choices and Take Purposeful Action

Depending upon your unique circumstances, there are any number of choices and actions that can be taken. It might take some time to identify all of them. I personally like list-making when I have problems that need to be solved. I will frequently share my list of choices with a friend or loved one, and sometimes that fresh pair of eyes will come up with a novel approach to the problem. Give yourself some time with this because, at the end of it all, you are really aiming to reaffirm purpose in your life (since work is such a big part of it!) and that is no small task. You never need to settle for anything that is making you feel compassion fatigued. Remember, it is *your* choice! The following are a few examples related to specific scenarios.

Possible choices and actions for dealing with incivility . . .

Perhaps it is that you have a coworker (or manager) who has been particularly nasty, bullying just about everyone on the unit, including yourself. Think about your options for handling the situation. The following are some suggestions of choices you can make (not meant to be all-inclusive; there are likely other possibilities unique to your situation):

- You can reach out and try to determine the underlying reason for your coworker's behavior.
- If you are not the only recipient of the bullying, you can choose to get everyone involved, by setting up a group meeting to discuss possible actions to take.
- You can choose to go to your superiors and inform them of the situation. (In taking the problem up the ladder, remember there is power in numbers!)
- You can choose to live and work with your coworker's bullying behavior. (Note, this is *not* a good choice!)
- You can choose to find an alternate place to work.

With the exception of the last choice listed, you actually have more than one choice. For example, you can reach out and try to get at the underlying reason for your coworker's behavior, and if that does not help to improve the situation, you can then go to your supervisor. If you are a nurse leader, you can explore each problem in the same manner. (Also see Chapter 11.)

Possible choices and actions for handling death overload . . .

Maybe you have witnessed too many patient deaths in the last few months. Think about your own situation. Writing down or sharing with others any sustaining memories you might have of experiences with dying and death can be helpful for healing.

Here are some suggestions of choices you can make (not meant to be all-inclusive):

- You can request critical incident stress debriefing.
- You can schedule some vacation time.
- You can see a grief counselor.
- You can request a transfer to a different area where dying and death occur less frequently.

Since there are so many things that might contribute to compassion fatigue, there will be lots of choices and purposeful actions that only you can identify, given your unique situation. Once you have figured out what choices you have depending upon your circumstances, you are ready to take action to begin to heal and to reaffirm purpose.

Step 3: Turn Outward Toward Self and Others

Stepping outside of yourself, turn toward yourself; look objectively at how you are caring for yourself. Do you make time for the important things? What *are* the important things for you? Consider your general health status, along with eating, sleeping, and maybe substance abuse patterns.

How are you interacting with others? Are you able to connect with your patients, loved ones, and coworkers? Seek support from friends and family—connect with them, talk about your feelings.

Some of the things you can do to reconnect with your own needs and with others include participating in meditation and yoga, attending specialized retreats and in-service education programs, and using employee assistance support services. (See the resource section for additional information.) Turn toward the things that make you smile— both little and big. It could be family, friends, pets, nature—a butterfly! Or if you prefer, music, art, a good book, a good movie; make time for the fun things.

Once you are on the path to healing you can try to prevent the reoccurrence (or minimize the occurrence) of compassion fatigue through mindful awareness. Pay attention to how you are living. One of the greatest gifts in my life was getting (and obviously surviving!) cancer—it continues to remind me how important it is to live each moment well. Journaling can be a very effective way to stay mindfully aware of our moments. Make some "me" time at the end of each day to jot down your thoughts, emotions, and any meaningful events that occurred. Make sure to note your feelings—the most potent indicator of when things might be off . . . or on!

KEY POINTS

- Compassion fatigue is a syndrome that occurs suddenly in response to a distressing or traumatic experience. It is relational in nature in that the compassion-fatigued individual is usually co-suffering with or internalizing the pain and anguish related to another.

- Trauma can be primary or secondary in nature; primary trauma is direct; for example, being mentally or physically hurt. Secondary trauma is when a person bears witness to another's suffering. What is and is not considered traumatic is highly individualized.
- Nurses are especially vulnerable to developing compassion fatigue because we are continually bearing witness to the suffering of others.
- The classic indication that one is experiencing compassion fatigue is feeling heart heavy and overburdened while continuing to do the work.
- Remaining connected to ourselves and our patients—being true to our authentic caring nature as nurses and remaining cognizant of the meaning and purpose of our work—can help to avert compassion fatigue.
- ART offers a framework to facilitate healing from compassion fatigue and may be helpful in thwarting its occurrence.

ENDNOTES

1. Vicarious trauma refers to a cumulative effect of witnessing the suffering of those who are traumatized, resulting in transformative changes in the carer; it is frequently noted to involve a loss of spiritual connection—feelings of hopelessness or helplessness.
2. Post-traumatic stress disorder results from being the recipient of and/or witnessing someone else experiencing primary trauma.
3. Emotional contagion refers to the idea that someone may "catch" and feel the emotions of another, similar to how one might "catch" a cold. In this manner, the emotions of individuals and groups of people can spread to others.
4. Negative subtle influences are referred to as active collusion functioning within automatisms (Briggs & Peat, 1999).

Chapter 7

I KNOW WHAT I OUGHT TO DO!

*Action may not always bring happiness, but there
is no happiness without action.*
—WILLIAM JAMES

*Our lives begin to end the day we become
silent about things that matter.*
—MARTIN LUTHER KING, JR.

KEY TOPICS

- Moral distress
- Unique professional knowledge
- The importance of nursing
- Moral courage

A re there things in your practice that you think ought to be done but feel
unable to do? Is the environment you are working in hindering rather
than enhancing your practice? Consider the following scenario:

> *Mrs. Frank is in the surgical intensive care unit after having had open
> heart surgery. In addition to the sternal surgical wound she has three
> chest tubes, a swan ganz, an arterial line, a femoral central line, and a
> foley. It is 86 degrees in the room and the nurse is perspiring as he
> works. He notices that the patient's dressings are coming off due to
> diaphoresis, and he attempts to reinforce them.*

> *The nurse knows that the patient is at risk for infection and that the
> environment is not conducive to healing. He feels helpless, for many
> times in the past he and other staff have reported the excessive heat*

on the unit to no avail, and in fact they had been told that there was nothing that could be done about it.

Mrs. Frank develops a high fever on her second postoperative day; the nurse wonders if it is because she is now septic and if the heat in the room may have contributed to the infection. He prays that the vancomycin they are starting will effectively treat the infection. At the end of the day he goes home worrying about his patient.

Does this sound familiar? Are there things in your practice that you know *ought* be different, but you feel at a loss to change?

DEFINING MORAL DISTRESS

Moral distress occurs "when one knows the right thing to do but institutional constraints make it nearly impossible to pursue the right course of action" (Jameton, 1984, p. 6). In essence, moral distress is a form of secondary trauma that over time can result in compassion fatigue and/or burnout. Moral distress can arise, like in the preceding clinical vignette, from any number of things in our practice environment. Corley (2002) identified that there are opposing internal and external factors involved: The nurse's values and sense of obligation (internal) can conflict with the values and views of an organization, other providers, patients, families, or even society (external).

Moral distress is also prevalent in nursing education, where faculty may find themselves in anguish for various reasons on behalf of students (Ganske, 2010). Nurse educators can contribute to moral distress in their students if they are not careful. A case in point is when a nurse faculty member tells her students that although they witnessed unsafe or substandard care in a clinical setting, because the students are students and they are all guests, they must not speak up about it.

The manifestations of moral distress are similar to those experienced by someone suffering from compassion fatigue. In fact, social worker Donna Forster (2009) has offered the idea that compassion fatigue may be more correctly understood as a *form* of moral stress. Unresolved or ongoing experiences of moral distress over time can result in burnout. The classic indication of moral distress is a sense of powerlessness due to feeling unable to carry out what one thinks is the right thing to do (Jameton, 1993). Anger, guilt, feeling unimportant or inadequate, difficulty sleeping, gastrointestinal upset, and any number of the multitude of signs and symptoms related to suffering can ensue.

THE BIGGEST CONTRIBUTING FACTOR

Nursing is predicated on a value for human life and on health and healing. It is through our service to, and connection with, others that we actualize our potential as nurses. Yet, many times nurses do *not* act the way they want to act or do what it is they know in their heart and mind needs to be done. In the current day literature, one reads how "nursing staff definitely appear to be experiencing moral frustration and guilt as a result of being prevented from providing the care they wish" (Schluter, Winch, Holzhauser, & Henderson, 2008, p. 318). I would point out that this has been the case for a pretty long time—it is nothing new. What I would like to know is why *we* have not been able to address the biggest contributor to moral distress in nursing, which, as far as I can tell, has always been either the nurse not being able to find (or use) his or her voice or, alternatively, working in a place where his or her voice does not seem to matter.

Many nurses cannot seem to make their voices heard. The reasons why this happens are many, but include our personal values and beliefs, our education (or lack thereof), our workplace, and the people who work with us. An overarching issue that crosses over all of it is the valuing and, conversely, devaluing of our unique nursing knowledge and skills.

When Our Voices Do Not Seem to Matter

In what today is deemed to be a classic, Roland Yarling and Beverly McElmurry (1986) expounded upon the importance of the moral foundation of our discipline as a determinant of our professional well-being. One of the most significant deterrents to doing what we know we *ought* to do continues to be what Yarling and McElmurry (1986) referred to as *hospitalonian captivity*. The health care systems in which we work put restrictions upon the profession, limiting what we can and cannot do, and our voices do not seem to matter. Accordingly, we often feel powerless. Their words were applicable a quarter of a century ago and remain so today:

> ... there is grave institutional culpability in a situation where the institutional disincentives to morally responsible action are so persuasive that the probability of moral action by the average person is rendered minimal ... nurses are not free to be moral because they are deprived of moral agency by the repressive character of the hospitals in which they practice. (p. 71)

There are definitely institutional disincentives that are worse than others. Take, for example, the case of the nurse who questioned a "doctor's orders" and was publicly reprimanded with a note on her locker door; that was pretty bad. But the nurse who is fired because she or he advocates for patients is much worse. There are other ways in which disincentives are covertly imposed. Having a heavy work load on a unit where patients often die does not encourage "presencing" for the nurse who feels compelled to be present with the patient and his or her loved ones. Instead, heavy workloads on these units deter nurses from doing what they feel they should be doing.

The Right to Have One's Part Matter

Nurses are not taught to be assertive, and without this skill it can be difficult to find one's voice or to make one be heard. Feminist and educator Carolyn Heilburn (1988) said that power is the "ability to take one's place in whatever discourse is necessary to action and the right to have one's part matter" (p. 18). Nurses in practice may frequently find themselves in a position where they feel as if their part does not matter at all. For instance, on the unit where the heat was excessive, not only were the patients suffering, the nurses that were providing care in that less than optimal environment were too. But none of the nurses felt that their voices were being heard—so they stopped using their voices completely about the issue.

In our code of ethics, Provision 6 emphasizes the part that we must play in cultivating an environment conducive to acting with ethical comportment (Fowler, 2008). Specifically, Provision 6.3 notes that "the nurse is responsible for contributing to a moral environment that encourages respectful interactions with colleagues, support of peers, and identification of issues that need to be addressed" (Fowler, 2008, p. 162). We also acknowledge in Provision 6.1 that the environment we work in can and does influence how we go about doing our work: "Both virtues and excellences, as aspects of moral character, can be either nurtured by the environment in which the nurse practices or they can be diminished or thwarted" (p. 161).

Recall the observations I shared earlier made by Liaschenko (2008), that her students—nurses engaged in practice—often felt their voices were not heard because *they* didn't know enough of the science. As a result, they believed that they were at fault for not being heard. Disturbingly, the relational aspects of nursing—the caring attributes—were not factored into their concerns at all (Liaschenko, 2008). At the end of the day, being dismissed by others as "noncredible knowers" was sufficient grounds for these nurses to *believe* themselves to *be* noncredible knowers.

Liaschenko (2008) emphasized that it is because nurses continue not to have the necessary freedom that enables them to speak up and act assertively to advocate on behalf of their patients, whereas others who work in health care have this freedom. While other health care professionals claim their legitimacy to speak up, assert that they are credible knowers, and insist on accountability from other members of the health care team, she noted that we in nursing do not. Liaschenko claimed that this is because we occupy a social space of "gendered labor" (p. 197), because care of the sick continues to be a predominantly female occupation, and because, well, even nurse educators often do not seem to value the caring aspects of the profession, which make us unique.

Not all nursing knowledge is considered "scientific," but it nevertheless has enormous value to facilitate health and healing. With our continued silence, inability to articulate what it is we do—choosing not to use our voices either because we are oppressed in our workplaces or because we believe we cannot or should not do so, we allow others to think that our contributions to health and healing are minimal, at best. *We* allow hospitalonian captivity to prevail.

PATTERNS OF KNOWING

We are not victims; we participate in creating reality through our actions. In essence, we give up the power we have as equal participants in assuring the quality of care received by our patients. We do this in large part by devaluing our unique ways of knowing. Nurse Barbara Carper (1978) identified patterns of knowing that are all important sources for knowledge acquisition: empirical, personal, ethical, and aesthetic. She noted that "each pattern may be conceived as necessary for achieving mastery in the discipline but none of them could be considered sufficient" (pp. 21–22). Empirical knowledge is the scientific component of nursing, based on empirics and evidence; personal knowledge arises from our self-understanding of who we are and how we feel; ethical knowledge is a matter of principles and codes, establishing what is right, and acting with moral comportment to do what one believes he or she ought to do; and aesthetic knowledge is the going beyond to seek meaning—it is fundamentally the artistic expression and comprehension of all that is and has yet to be (Carper, 1978).

Focusing solely on empirical ways of knowing—scientific knowledge—does not take into account the human characteristic of uniqueness. It is surely a cause for concern when we follow "standing orders" or "clinical pathways" without taking into account the distinct variability from one person to another. We always have outliers and everyone wonders what *we* are doing wrong. What is wrong is that the health care system is emphasizing one way of knowing—empirics—and not using any of the others (personal, ethical, aesthetic). Needless to say, none of the patterns of knowing can stand alone without becoming less effective. As nurse Christopher Johns (1995) noted:

> Whereas empirics encourages the practitioner to stereotype the situation according to some rule or law that predicts an outcome, aesthetic knowing involves a process of perceiving or grasping the nature of a clinical situation; interpreting this information in order to understand its meaning for those involved, whilst envisioning desired outcomes in order to respond with appropriate and skilled action, and subsequently reflecting on whether the outcomes were effectively achieved. (p. 228)

All of our ways of knowing combine to *complete us* as nurses.

The tragedy is that most nurses are not educated to believe in our inherent value and the contributions that all of our unique ways of knowing make to human health and healing. On more than one occasion, I have heard fellow colleagues as well as other health care professionals say that nurses were and always will be handmaidens to physicians. I have never believed myself to be that, and I do not educate "would-be nurses" to believe it either. Nevertheless, the image of the handmaiden is, without a doubt, reinforced through our language and social practices, such as is evident in the story of "doctor's orders" I shared earlier.

CHOICE AND POWER: DEVELOPING A SENSE OF OUR OWN SALIENCE

That it is a choice nurses make (to value some ways of knowing and skills more than others) is obvious, but our choices are often influenced, and then reinforced, by others. Take, for example, a nurse practitioner (NP) who is purportedly in collaborative practice or is functioning as an independent practitioner. She is told that she must limit her time with patients to 15 minutes each visit; however, she knows that some patients require more time, others less. Still, she may choose to conform rather than say this to her administrators or the physicians she is in practice with, or perhaps she does share her concern but it is not valued.

The NP's practice is changed based on the influence of others or the policies of the institution rather than her getting the system to accommodate her practice the way she knows it should be. More than likely, she probably feels she has no choice in the matter. One might say that the NP does not have a choice, and perhaps the individual NP does not, for if she refuses she may well find herself out of a job. But collectively, NPs *do* have a choice—it is, after all, their patients, their practice, their licenses, and it is also their right to have "their part matter."

Some may think this is a simplistic view of a complex problem and I might agree, if it were not for the fact that people who do not understand what nursing entails are making the rules for things like this in our practice and I know that many of our physician colleagues agree. An NP is not supposed to function like an MD; they are different roles. Certainly there is overlap because both are primary care providers; however, nurses look at wholes, physicians (usually), specific parts. The two roles should complement one another.

Although I used the NP as an example, I want to stress that bedside nurses, nurse leaders, clinical nurse specialists (CNSs), and even nurse educators, are all influenced by others and by the policies and procedures in our workplaces. If we are allowing others to make decisions concerning our profession and practice, it is ultimately still a choice that *we* are making.

In one of my stints as a CNS, I wanted to be on the hospital Pharmacy and Therapeutics Committee. I was the only CNS in the entire hospital, a large teaching hospital, and I thought I belonged there, but the deputy director of nursing, who I answered directly to, said that the "big boys club" would not want a nurse there; for the same reason I was told that I couldn't be the team leader of a CQI project that I initiated. I had to ask a physician to be the leader, even though he rarely came to meetings and I did all of the work. I realized it was still my choice and that perhaps the effort I was making—coming in the back door, so to speak up—was effective, to a point. But I also recognized that it was to some degree a new take on an old game, a game that nurses have played in some fashion for decades: treading lightly, saying to the MD, "Do you think perhaps that this might be a better way?" Instead of saying bluntly, *"This is a better way."*

With little things, it might be ok to play that game, but with the bigger things, it is never ok because it leads us to moral distress. Over time, and especially with repeated occurrences, moral residue builds—long-lasting effects that are very hard to shake (Webster & Bayliss, 2000). We are wounded in such a way that our sense of self is compromised. Our moral concerns have not been acknowledged—we have not been acknowledged—and we begin to believe that our voices really do not matter.

Nurse scholar and practitioner Elizabeth Ann Manhart Barrett (1989, 2010) stresses that everyone has power, it is just a matter of how we go about actualizing it. She noted that there are two ways to view *power*, similar to my claim about two views of energy: Power can be defined and actualized as control or as knowing participation (Barrett, 2010). *Power as control* is the normal way many people go about influencing change. It is predicated on domination over others and other things, whereas *power as knowing participation* entails a person's awareness, choices, freedom to choose, and involvement in creating change (Barrett,

1989, 2010). We have to be aware that we have choices we can make, and then we must feel free to choose and be involved in creating change.

In nursing, many of us have been conditioned to allow *power as control* to suppress us and devalue our very real power as the largest constituent of professionals in health care. It is through our knowing participation as compassionate, competent carers that people are able to actualize their potentials to live well and die well. That is *real power*—we have it, but we do not exercise it as well as we should, perhaps because many of us are kept un-blissfully ignorant (unaware!) by the way we have been taught. It is time to change all that. As Shirley MacLaine (2011) notes in her latest writings, it is time for each of us to reiterate, "I am all over that." Try saying, I am over being oppressed, being made to feel subordinate, being told to do what I know I shouldn't do, and being prevented from doing what I know I ought to do. It is time to *know* our power and to live it together.

Pat Benner and colleagues (Benner, Sutphen, Leonard, Day, & Shulman 2009) wrote about the transformation needed in nursing education if we are to keep up with the fast pace of health care, stressing the widening gap between education and practice. They emphasized that nurses have to develop a sense of salience; that practitioners must be able to identify what is and isn't important in terms of clinical priorities. But in cases where nurses experience moral distress, it is usually not due to not having a sense of what the priorities are; quite on the contrary, it often appears to be just the opposite. We *know* what we are supposed to do, we know what appears to be the right thing to do, yet we feel unable to do it. Thus, it is equally important for nurses to develop a sense of our *own* salience.

At the onset of our careers, we should be taught that what we do is enormously important and that the actions we take, both little and large, make a difference in the quality of people's living-dying. To have a sense of what is and isn't important will not do much for the nurse who cannot make her voice heard. Note that it is not too late to develop a sense of your own salience. The following is an AHA! shared by an RN in one of my classes:

> *To narrow my experience during this course of when I came to the realization of some meaning or understanding that I did not have before is difficult because of the many things that we covered and learned; however, it was during one session that the professor had the class complete a survey which is used to assess burnout, when I came to an epiphany that, although I was close to burnout, I did not want to be like those nurses who exhibit all the signs of burnout. During this class discussion, the professor, possibly without knowing, helped me come to the realization that, although I enjoy*

working with the mentally ill, the program I am working at may not be where I want to continue working.

For some time I had been sharing my concerns about patients' medication responses with the program psychiatrist, and I felt like I hit a brick wall when I went to administration to further address the issue. I continued to witness patients demonstrating severe side effects from the psychotropic medications being administered to them. Their medications were not being monitored properly, and some patients were on unnecessarily high dosages that more than likely contributed to the worsening of their conditions. While this is not an end-of-life situation, it does contribute to the quality of life of patients and reflects the ethical decisions that nurses have to deal with in the work place . . . . This class made me realize that, although I am not in complete control of what is happening in the place where I work, my enthusiasm and concern for the patients, as a nurse, and my efforts to expand my education in the field have an impact that is important and makes a difference.

This student was in a workplace where he was experiencing moral distress on a daily basis; coming back to school was the best thing for him and for his patients—what he learned empowered him and over time he was able to develop a sense of his own importance.

Assert Yourself! You Have a Right to be Heard

My favorite nurse author on the subject of assertiveness is Melodie Chenevert (1988), who noted that nurses have a collective goal: "We want to make safe, sane, humane health care available" (p. x). She stressed that assertiveness might be the most significant skill for nurses to learn in order to achieve that goal. I agree. Over the years I have often wondered, where does one learn this important skill? It is obvious that most nurses do not get assertiveness training while in school. In fact, Chenevert's wonderful books on assertiveness training are out of print; I emailed her trying to get her to have them republished. It amazes and disgruntles me that, over 30 years later, her words are still so applicable to us in nursing. Find a copy of one or two; you will be equally amazed and disgruntled and you will learn an awful lot in a short space of time, I promise you.

Not meaning to be sexist, I must nevertheless point out the obvious (which Chenevert also pointed out): Nursing is a predominantly female profession and with it comes some very real issues. That is why throughout this book, I most often refer to the nurse as a "she," not to be stereotypical or to leave out the men in our profession, rather, just to be realistic . . . We are MOSTLY women. Not every cultural tradition holds the belief that women are equal to men, and even when it is believed that this is so, not every woman is treated equally and not every woman *expects* to be treated equally.

Carol Gilligan (1982), in her groundbreaking work on the voices of women in moral decision making, noted the following:

> As we have listened for centuries to the voices of men and the theories of development that their experience informs, so we have come more recently to notice not only the silence of women but the difficulty in hearing what they say when they speak up. Yet in the different voice of women lies the truth of an ethic of care, the tie between relationship and responsibility, and the origins of aggression in the failure of connection. (p. 173)

When nurses—predominantly women—are prevented from valuing the connection to self and other, the caring practices inherent in our work, it is not good for us individually or collectively.

The basic premise underlying assertiveness training is that we have a right to be heard and respected as human beings. But, in order to *learn* assertiveness, we first have to believe in ourselves; we each have to turn toward the mirror and recognize our own inherent value as a person and as a professional. Because to assert oneself means, for all intents and purposes, to communicate one's opinions, values, and beliefs in such a way that others take notice, but not in such as way that it is viewed as an act of aggression. Without a sense of our own salience, we may not believe our own opinion should count and, thus, we will not assert ourselves. We will not bother to try to make our voices heard.

I was fortunate in that, early on in my career, I had an incredible nurse educator named Judy Carlson-Catalano for a nursing leadership course in my Bachelor of Science in Nursing (BSN) program (I am a firm believer in giving credit where it is due!). I took the course while I was working as a fairly new RN, having graduated not too long before from an Associate Degree (AD) program, and I was already unhappy with some of the things I saw and experienced at work. She introduced us to Chenevert and she taught us how important we were. Judy stressed that we had power—power in numbers, intelligence, and caring. It was she who talked me out of going to law school when I completed my BSN, a decision that I have never regretted. Have you ever had an educator like this one? If so, then you must already have a sense of your own salience; if not, than now is a good time to learn some of the things we were taught in that class.

With wit and clarity, Chenevert (1988) asked us in her book *STAT: Special Techniques in Assertiveness Training for Women in the Health Professions*, who we would choose to be—chickens or eagles. She claimed that many of us are eagles with a chicken complex. We do not realize that we can fly; we can soar above the trees. Instead, we believe what we have been conditioned to believe, and for nurses, especially those who are women, we have been conditioned in various ways to believe that we answer to others and that our jobs consist of following "orders." Like Chenevert (1988) noted, we may think we belong in a barnyard eating chicken feed, rather than using our eagle gifts—powers of flight and keen vision.

I always point out to my students that getting into nursing school is no easy task. Staying in nursing school is even less so. It takes intelligence, courage, perseverance, compassion, and incredible skill to be a nurse. We really are *wonderful* people; we should love and respect ourselves, each other, and our important contributions to the health care world.

What happens when we do have a sense of our own salience but others do not? When we use our voice and it is not heard? If we are working in a system where this repeatedly occurs, we may well find ourselves losing our voice—or at least no longer choosing to use it. We may begin to doubt ourselves and our importance as the moral residue builds. Or we can stand up and fight, like the two nurse administrators did in Texas, who then found themselves fired for reporting a physician who was practicing "bad medicine" (Sack, 2010).

It Is not Whistle-Blowing, It Is Advocacy!

Ann Mitchell and Vickilyn Galle, both nurses working as administrators in quality improvement and who had worked a combined 47 years at their hospital, began trying to get the attention of hospital administration in 2008 related to the patient care practices of a particular physician, which were clearly a cause for apprehension (Sack, 2010). Their worries fell on deaf ears and they then turned to other measures to protect the patients—sending off an unsigned letter to the Texas Medical Board detailing their concerns.

When it was discovered that it was Mitchell and Galle who had sent the letter, both nurses were fired. Adding insult to injury, they were then indicted and threatened with 10 years in prison for misuse of official information, a third-degree felony in the state of Texas (Sack, 2010). Galle was acquitted shortly afterward, and when Mitchell went to trial, she too was acquitted. Both vindicated, they filed a civil suit and were ultimately awarded $750,000 to be shared between them. But no amount of money could rectify this wrong.

What did the hospital administrators hope to accomplish by firing these nurses? How might the fear of negative consequences such as this deter other nurses (and would-be nurses) from acting with moral comportment? No matter how you look at it, the entire thing was bad news for everyone.

Whistle-blowers are supposed to be protected for reporting to the authorities' bad practices and conditions that put people, and on occasion, other living things, in harm's way; however, I take offense when nurses who act with moral comportment are called "whistle-blowers." A well-meaning person might make a phone call to the authorities concerning the practices of a group of people who are cutting down trees in a forest, damaging an ecologic environment that is supposed to be protected; that is considered whistle-blowing. An office worker who calls the state environmental protection agency because he finds there is uncontained asbestos in the office ceiling and finds out that his employer has been hiding the risk from all of the office workers; that is whistle-blowing. On the other hand, nurses are patient carers and advocates; we are not whistle-blowers. We are the *first* and *last* line of defense for people who are very often vulnerable and who put their complete trust in us to compassionately, competently, care for *and* protect them. In fact, the public routinely votes the nursing profession as one of the most trusted; we are *expected* to speak up!

Just as I am writing this, the annual Gallup poll report has been released, indicating that the public once again ranked nurses to be the most trustworthy and ethical of all groups (Jones, 2011). If we do *not* act to protect, then that line of defense is broken and we might as well throw up a white flag, surrendering our moral code along with the values and excellences deemed to be the foundational core of our profession. And that is what eventually happens when we know what we ought to do but are repeatedly unable to do it. The result: moral distress → moral residue → burnout.

When We Are the Cause of Anguish

Suffering is an ineluctable part of living and dying; however, many times we in health care unintentionally cause further anguish through our acts. We not only bear witness to suffering but sometimes also directly cause what is clearly unnecessary suffering. When this occurs repeatedly, we find ourselves wondering what the goals of care are, and over time, we may well find ourselves flicking the shutoff switch to the anguish in our patients' eyes. It could be what seems on the surface to be a simple matter, like bed scale weights or even little things like taking rectal temperatures in cardiac critical care, because it is considered the most accurate thing to do. How many men do you know whose heart rate would not increase when told to lie on their side so you could take a rectal temperature? Well, I remember a coworker's story of taking a rectal temperature on a male patient who went into v-tachycardia during the procedure; she did a precordial thump, which luckily converted his rhythm. Imagine the possibility of losing a patient because you asked him to turn over to get a rectal temperature? Of course we can laugh about it now, only because we no longer do rectal temperatures . . . but I bet many nurses can think of a thing or two that is being done in their practice, which they are not laughing about, knowing that it may be causing more harm than good.

One of the common practices that really irks me in teaching hospitals is when patients are used by interns and residents for learning how to do things such as line insertions—the day before, and the morning of, surgery. Some of these patients are going for very risky procedures, and some of them are going to die. Yet they spend their last day or so as pin cushions and guinea pigs for those who are there to learn, separated from their loved ones in the process. Where is the beneficence in that?

Unfortunately, it seems that many interns and residents who are learning how to do things (on patients) have already distanced themselves so much that they do not recognize the human beings they are oftentimes literally torturing with their unskilled hands. When I was in practice, I frequently advocated for patients to be left alone after the first stick or two and insisted an experienced nurse or physician come in to do the sticking. In the last decade I have had many occasions where I have witnessed these kinds of occurrences with loved ones (and on occasion even myself) and have wondered, "Where is the nurse?" (I return to this question again later.)

On medical surgical and oncology units, nurses are frequently faced with knowing that a patient is scheduled for diagnostic tests or procedures that will not improve his or her quality of life and which may in fact create unnecessary suffering. For instance, I remember assigning a student to work with an older adult who had recently been diagnosed with stage 3b lung cancer. He was admitted for uncontrollable diarrhea and diagnosed with *Clostridium difficile* colitis (*C. diff*).

Speaking with him about his choices, he shared some personal information. He was estranged from most of his family; he had eight grown children and was not sure how many grandchildren he had. He lived alone and rarely saw anyone. He said he had made some bad choices as a youngster— he "loved to drink and he loved the women." Now, he was ready to die, he said, and he opted not to receive any treatment for his late-stage cancer. He made that very clear. His plan was to return home as soon as his diarrhea was resolved. The following week when we returned to the unit, this man was being sent for radiation therapy. When asked why, he told me and the student that the MD said he had to have the treatment.

Another time, when I was working as a nursing supervisor, we had an increased incidence of postoperative infections in the cardiothoracic surgical intensive care unit. In retrospect, it was found that the staff and many of the advanced practice nurses knew what the likely cause was; several of the surgical interns and residents were not washing their hands when they were taking down and changing dressings. Yet no one had documented or acted on it. It was not until the State came in that the problem became general knowledge and was rectified. At a staff meeting a few weeks later, many of the nurses voiced having felt morally distressed about it but none of them had had the moral courage to come forward.

As an educator, I look around and I say it is no wonder. I do not see us in nursing education spending anywhere near enough time teaching our students how important *they* are and how to use their voices; rather, I see extraordinary emphasis being placed on clinical skill development.

What Do You Mean I Am Not Allowed to Be Sick?

Nussbaum (1996) pointed out that a concern for the good of others often leads one to risk his or her own contentment: "For people very often sacrifice their own interests and well-being, and in many cases even their own lives, for the well-being of those they love, or for good social consequences that they prize" (p. 49). Nurses are self-sacrificing; we go in to work when physically or emotionally exhausted (like I did when returning a fourth night to care for John Doe), we skip breaks and meals, we stay long after our shift ends to complete various tasks, and so forth. We will go to great lengths to get what our patients need, wearing ourselves out completely in the process.

We have been conditioned to sacrifice our own interests and well-being. We are informed that we must not call in sick and that our patients and unit duties come before our own needs. Even while in nursing education, the expectation is that we will not miss classes, and, consequently, students frequently drag themselves into classes sick and expose everyone else to illness. Heck, I had an emergency C-section during my senior year in nursing school and signed out against medical orders, running a temperature no less, to go to my clinical because I was certain the instructor would not allow me to pass the course if I missed it. Why did I feel that way? Because it was emphasized repeatedly that we could not miss any clinical days (and my professor showed no compassion whatsoever).

When we are conditioned for unfair expectations it leads to moral distress, because we are then torn between doing what we have always been told is the right thing versus what we intuit is needed for our own well-being. If we act in our own best interests, for example, calling in sick, we chance feeling guilty because we left our unit short of staff. We perceive ourselves as the cause or contributor of another's anguish.

ACTING WITH MORAL COURAGE VERSUS
FEELING POWERLESS

There is another side to the self-sacrificing nurse. There is the nurse, who literally lays him- or herself on the line in order to advocate for others. This is the nurse who is said to have moral courage, the one who acts with moral comportment, regardless of risk to his or her own well-being. There are plenty of nurses who have a great deal of moral courage, and there would undoubtedly be more if all nurses had a sense of their own salience. Make no mistake; I am not slapping anyone's wrist here on this issue, either. It is difficult to have moral courage if you have no awareness of your own power and no confidence in your own ability. It is difficult to have moral courage in an organization that does not support it. Without a just culture, most people will not be particularly courageous about anything.

Nurse educators and leaders can encourage the development of moral courage in their students and staff, if they emulate it themselves. The nurse educator is the gatekeeper for the profession and the developer of future nursing practice. The nurse leader who supports and fosters quality caring ultimately sets the tone for a healthy work environment (Edmonson, 2010). That is why nurse educators and leaders need to be cultivated in an atmosphere where, as Barrett's (2010) power theory demarcates, *power as knowing participation* is stressed and where *power as control* is minimized. We need transformational leaders and transformational educators (see Chapter 11).

APPLYING ART FOR MORAL DISTRESS

To address moral distress on an individual basis one needs to first acknowledge if there is a problem getting one's voice to be heard. However, acknowledging and making known to others our worth as nurses who contribute so much to health and healing and whose voices do matter is a task for *all* nurses, including leaders and educators. We must first recognize the importance of the profession as a whole. We need to turn toward ourselves by teaching and learning how to insist that our voices do matter and toward others in how we approach the care of our patients, to act with assertion—with moral comportment and courage—to do what we believe is right and what is needed.

Step 1: Acknowledge a Feeling or Wound That Needs Healing

Can you think of any regular practices that bother you because you think you should or should not be doing them? Or perhaps there are things that used to bother you and you are no longer paying attention to them or have given up trying to change your practice? A case in point is the nurse who knows that it is too warm on the unit but no longer asks for the temperature control to be fixed; or the nurse who continues to do bed scale weights, simply because it was "ordered," all the while knowing it may cause additional suffering; or the nurse who knows that another course of chemotherapy is not going to make things better, yet when the patient asks about it, she feels that she cannot speak up. As you go about your work, identify any uncomfortable feelings—capture your moments by writing them down so that you can reflect upon them later.

Step 2: Recognize Choices and Take Purposeful Action

If you are experiencing moral distress, depending upon the circumstances, you will have any number of choices. In addition to the specifics of each case, you need to reflect upon your

- Values and beliefs
- Relationships with the people with whom you work
- Support systems

Ask yourself, in light of these, what choices you have that might make things better for you and for your patients. List them.

1. _____
2. _____
3. _____
4. _____
5. _____

Who might listen to your concerns and support you in making the necessary changes in practice? Can you approach your administrative staff alone or do you need the support of coworkers? If there is an ethics committee in your institution, you can certainly approach them. If not, maybe you can seek support outside of your institution; such has regularly been the case with students who contact me after graduation to help them brainstorm ways to address concerns in their practice. Or perhaps you need to take a more radical action like the nurses who contacted the medical board about unsafe medical practices or the nurse who calls in the State for an unsafe environment.

When working as a clinical specialist in a fairly large teaching hospital, there was a period of time when there was a string of medication errors on several medical surgical units. Consequently, as is often the case, the staff nurses were being disciplined and in-serviced to no end. The morale on the units was low and nurses were scared. Some of the staff spoke with me; one told me she was looking for a new job and another said she was going back to school. I went home each night troubled and spent hours talking about the problem with my husband. It was one of the times I lost sleep over work.

On further exploration of the issue, during which time I did a retrospective study of the patient charts, physician prescriptions, and incident reports, I found that it was actually the physicians who needed in-service education regarding how they were writing the prescriptions. The majority of the nurses knew there was a problem and, in fact, a few had taken it upon themselves to just change the scripts, which of course is beyond a staff nurse's scope of practice. What the staff nurses really needed was not in-servicing on medication errors, but rather assertiveness training in order to be able to go back to the physician and say, "No, this is not right."

If you do not feel an issue can be addressed by yourself or you are unable to direct the issue to the appropriate person and there does not seem to be anywhere to turn for support, you still have choices to make. You can choose to advocate, climbing the ladder up, and mayhap not just up but also out (such as the nurse administrators who reported the physician to the medical board in Texas) until your voice has been heard. Or, if you do not see that happening, maybe it is time to move on. Weigh your choices. If you are being repeatedly put in a position where your license or health might be in jeopardy and there is nothing else you can do to make things better, start to look around for a new position. The one thing we must not do is settle; we must never choose to compromise our beliefs and values. We must never flick the shutoff switch. When the switch is flicked off, the bad is becoming ugly!

If you are unable to find your voice, another choice you have is to seek assertiveness training. There are training programs available (see the resource section for further information or just Google it). I mentioned earlier Melodie Chenevert's writings on the subject, she has written a number of helpful exercises that can be used individually or in group sessions. When I worked as a clinical nurse manager, I adopted one for use with staff and it was a big hit (I will come back to this in Chapter 11).

Step 3: Turn Outward Toward Self and Others

In patient cases leading to moral distress, it can be helpful to ask yourself what your beliefs and values are, and then where possible, try to explore all sides of the situation. This is important because, in any given situation, others may or may not feel the same way that you do. If you can, speak with others about the issue. In the classes where I teach ethics, I frequently ask that the students dialogue in a special way put forward by physicist David Bohm (1996), where all participants must make an effort to hear one another's viewpoint. As per Bohm's basic principles on dialogue, I emphasize that we are not trying to drive the conversation in any way or to any specific conclusions; thus, we must agree to suspend individual judgment during our discussions, remaining open and honest. In this way we can try to build upon one another's ideas. The end result is always that individual perspectives shift and one's beliefs and values sometimes change completely.

I have used Bohm's dialogue method in a number of classes, most notably in graduate-level bioethics courses. The majority of students in these classes are seasoned nurses, some who have been working for decades. The stories they share during our dialogues related to ethical dilemmas they have faced in practice indicate that moral distress can linger and fester over time. Some of these nurses noted that they never felt there was an opportunity to talk about their concerns; consequently, they had internalized their anguish. Sharing their stories in class, and having time to reflect upon and dialogue with others about them, was a healing experience.

When discussing ethical issues, in particular, the nature of the topics is such that no discussion can yield an understanding of the human race at large; there are far too many different beliefs on life, living, death, dying, health, and healing. By understanding that the view from the looking glass can vary considerably from person to person, we can come to see the world anew, perhaps unlearning or relearning long-held beliefs, values, and ideas.

Once you have explored your feelings in relation to other points of view, if your perspective does not shift, and it is making you feel helpless and/or ineffective, and you believe it is affecting patients, their loved ones, coworkers, or perchance even your loved ones, it is time to act. Think: The choices I make can change how I feel, how my patients heal, how my colleagues work together, how I interact with loved ones. Reconnect, now. As Henry David Thoreau noted, "Only that day dawns to which we are awake."

When moral distress occurs in health care, it is usually a group-level happening so that turning outward toward self and others may be especially effective in group sessions. Clinical leaders and educators can try taking a specific situation and explore it from a group perspective. On occasion, it might be fitting to encourage discourse by taking it out of the unit or current moment of moral distress. I like to use short clips of events (such as those from the motion picture *Wit* or *Patch Adams*) to encourage dialogue about critical issues.

The American Association of Critical Care Nurses (2006) has put forward a model called "The 4 A's to Rise Above Moral Distress" created by their ethics work group. The four A's stand for "Ask, Affirm, Assess, and Act," and as a whole, they offer a framework to address moral distress in the workplace. Check out the resource section at the end of the book to learn more.

KEY POINTS

- Moral distress arises when you know what the right thing to do is in a given situation, but feel for whatever reason unable to do it.

- Moral distress can occur from conflicts related to our own personal values and beliefs, surfacing in the many ethical dilemmas we face, as well as from interpersonal discord between coworkers or members of the health care team, patients, and their families, or it can be related to environmental factors that we know are not conducive to health and healing.

- The biggest contributing factor to moral distress in nursing is nurses feeling, or being, unable to make their voice heard.

- Repeated instances of moral distress lead to the buildup of moral residue and over time can result in burnout.

- Developing a sense of our own salience as nurses individually and collectively so that we feel we have not only the responsibility but the right to speak up can help to prevent repeated instances of moral distress.

- Assertiveness skills can be developed in order to learn how to effectively use one's voice. We have a right to be heard!

- Self-reflection as well as group-level discussion of uncontrollable events that lead to moral distress can facilitate a converging of viewpoints and, in cases where that may not be possible, it can still help everyone to be more aware and participate more knowingly in changes that will benefit everyone.

Chapter 8

BURNT OUT AND SEEMINGLY HEARTLESS

I suffer from nothing. I no longer know what
suffering is. I have come to an end of all that . . . .
—GRAHAM GREENE

KEY TOPICS

- Burnout
- Consequences for nurses and patients

In his 1960 book, *A Burnt-Out Case*, novelist Graham Greene described his protagonist, a famous male architect named Querry, who, having become disillusioned with his work and life, chooses to disappear into the African jungle. There he takes on work in a colony with lepers and, in so doing, transforms his life in positive ways. The term *burnt-out case* refers to a leper whose disease has eaten away until it no longer exists and is consequently considered at the point of cure. But by that time, many lepers are missing limbs. In this story it is clear that the protagonist himself is a burnt-out case, although he suffers not from leprosy but from apathy. Instead of missing limbs, Querry seems numb and heartless.

A more complete idea of burnout as job stress arose in the 1970s and today it is recognized as a global phenomenon that is of significance due to the negative changes that result from it in both people and their workplace environments (Schaufeli, Leiter, & Maslach, 2009). Despite the noteworthy implications of burnout, there continues to be wide variation in terms of how it is defined, what contributes to the manifestation of it, how to treat it, and how to prevent it. In some countries, for instance, *burnout* is an actual medical diagnosis, while in others it is a nonmedical label (Schaufeli et al., 2009). Imagine being able to legitimately call in sick with a diagnosis of burnout!

The term burnout really caught on as an acute form of job stress when a psychiatrist equated the emotional exhaustion and loss of commitment he and others experienced in their work with the lasting effects of chronic drug abuse exhibited in drug abusers (Freudenberger, 1975). Around the same period, a social psychologist, Christina Maslach (1976, 1982), was studying the emotions of individuals who worked in human services. In her interviews with people, many voiced feeling emotionally exhausted, had negative feelings about their patients and coworkers, and questioned their own abilities as professionals. They referred to what they were feeling as "burnout," and many of them identified it with feelings of energy depletion, hence, the idea that one is "running on empty."

While the bulk of early studies focused on burnout in the caring professions, research later extended into all kinds of workplaces and we now know that one does not have to be in a caring profession to experience burnout. As of 2009, it was estimated that there were over 6,000 publications on the topic, and a countless number of studies have been performed and healing strategies developed to address the syndrome (Schaufeli et al., 2009).

DEFINING BURNOUT

Burnout is a broad-based syndrome that develops gradually as a person interacts with his or her workplace: "When the workplace does not recognize the human side of work or demands superhuman efforts, people feel overloaded, frustrated, and well, burned out" (Maslach & Leiter, 1999, p. 50). It can also be associated with an imbalance of demand and resources along with the fact that the ideal and the real often differ to the extent that one is frequently chasing rainbows that dissipate when approached. Burned out people feel hopeless to create change, and so over time they flick a shutoff switch.

Disenchanted and Disillusioned

In a way, burnout is a widespread disenchantment with one's work. Karl Emil Maximilian Weber (known as Max Weber; 1958), a German sociologist and political economist, discussed the concept of *disenchantment* as the manifestation of a generalized devaluing of beliefs accompanied by an increased valuing of scientific rationalization in modernity. Sadly, it often seems that this is what we are doing in both nursing education and practice. We are devaluing our core values and beliefs while elevating the scientific knowledge base of nursing. On another level, I suppose one could equate disenchantment with dehumanization, for when you remove the subjective and replace it with only objective, you remove most of what makes us uniquely human. Disenchantment is sometimes equated with disillusionment, a rude awakening of sorts where one is faced with a reality that is less than ideal.

When we are enchanted, we are enamored with something—we value it as something worthwhile. We are more apt to be engaged, interested, and motivated because we like whatever it is we are doing or are "enchanted with." Conversely, when we are disenchanted, we are more likely to be disengaged, disinterested, and unmotivated. We are emotionally empty—heart empty—and suffer with a generalized apathy. It is a form of suffering that transforms our very being into an almost *non-being* kind of existence. It is when we become routinely robotic!

Of all the professions, nursing is the one that has been most studied in relation to the phenomenon of burnout. Why is that the case? Because there are so many things inherent in the profession that set us up for burnout—we are the people most at risk to develop it!

WHAT STACKS THE DECK FOR NURSES TO BURN OUT?

To list the things that put the odds in our favor, I will reiterate the obvious. We have been, and continue to be, a predominantly female profession and, as I already noted, women are *not* equal to men in all cultures and environments.

Women remain the predominant carers in the home for loved ones, where there often is unequal work distribution related to household responsibilities. Like Chenevert (1988) noted, "While today's women are expected to bring home the bacon, today's men are still not expected to fry it" (p. 124). A case in point is the too-frequent occasion when I arrive home at 9 p.m., after putting in a 16-hour day, and my husband will tell me he has not eaten dinner. I might respond that I have not had a moment to go to the bathroom let alone eat a meal and that I ate Twinkies for breakfast, lunch, and dinner. His typical response will be something along the lines of, "You could call for a pizza." Geez, he is doing me a favor ... I do not have to cook! To be fair, I did choose to work at a university several hours away from home—that is not his fault. But surely there is something lop-sided here—just once couldn't he cook or at least called for the pizza?!

Pecking Orders Prevail ...

Physicians continue to be predominantly male, and this is at least partly responsible for why there seems to be a natural pecking order that goes from them to us. The "physician's order" mentality prevails in academia, practice, and also policy. A case in point is the advent of the *Physicians Order for Life Sustaining Treatment* (POLST). In some states, advanced practice nurses (APNs) and other health care professionals may also use the POLST forms. Yet, they are labeled a "physician's order." To give credit where due, it should be noted that some areas are a bit more diplomatic (less paternalistic) about it and refer to the form as the *Medical Order for Life Sustaining Treatment* (MOLST). The point is, with the continued use of expressions of paternalism comes a message that the physician is the superior.

Who gets paid better, the physician or the nurse? Who works better hours and is able to, for the most part, choose which days can be taken off for play? And, who seems to be more respected by others both in and out of health care settings? For example, it is puzzling that we have so many incredible nurses with much to impart to others and who speak so eloquently, and yet there have been major nursing conferences where physicians were the keynote speakers . . . conversely, I have yet to hear of a nurse being a keynote speaker at a major medical conference. Why is that? I definitely do not have an answer. When nurses become regular keynote speakers at physician events, it will be a sure sign that something has fundamentally changed for the better in terms of nurses being valued as full partners.

Please do not think that I am making this all about the male–female disparities that continue to be prominent in all business sectors, including academia, where it is well known that women do not get paid as much or advance as quickly as men. Do male nurses suffer from compassion fatigue and burnout? Absolutely! But many of the issues that prevail in nursing do so because of the male–female thing, the gender inequity that persists both overtly and covertly. Virginia Valian, professor of psychology and linguistics at Hunter College and the Graduate Center of City University of New York, has studied and written quite a lot about the subject. She pointed out that women continue to make less money and advance more slowly in *every* field, *including nursing* (Valian, 2006).

I am not necessarily advocating that nurses need to earn more money; clearly the economics of the health care system is such that in order to pay higher salaries one would have to decrease the number of nurses who work in the health care system, and that would only make things worse. What I am emphasizing is that wherever there is inequitable distribution of rewards *and* respect, there is bound to be an unhappy workforce. Society in general places higher accord to those who earn better salaries. Why this is the case has never made much sense to me. Perhaps it is because those who earn more seem to have more (from a materialistic point of view, anyway). Nevertheless, most nurses didn't go into nursing because of the amount of money that we could earn, or the material things we could buy, for surely, if one can become a nurse, *one could become most anything else*.

Burnout is said to be the result of cumulative frustration with one's workplace environment, and for nurses, many of the things that contribute to our frustration are more relational in nature than anything else. They have to do with whom we work (both patients and coworkers), how we interact with each other, and whether we are respected and valued for what it is we do. Far too often, our interpersonal relationships at work are less than satisfactory. A number of factors feed into this as well, including status and role incongruities, different personalities, organizational structure, and obviously, leadership styles.

Since a lot of the things nurses do are not valued, many who began their careers as very compassionate, competent carers, over time seem to value less the caring aspects of their own work. It is then that the technical skills and the lab values might become more important than the human-to-human connection. I think of this as *disenchantment in action*. The purported science of nursing becomes more important than the art of nursing, and, as a result, the science of nursing becomes more visible, while the art of nursing is discernibly less visible and in some cases seems to disappear altogether. When that occurs, with it comes burnout.

Nursing Education

Our nursing education helps us stack the deck against ourselves, not only by often accentuating what is deemed the science of nursing while minimizing the art of nursing (for lack of a better term to denote the caring relational aspects of our practice) in our basic education but also because we continue to have multiple entry levels into practice. With diploma, AD, BS, MS, and doctoral level entry programs, and then all the certificate programs, it really is difficult for people to understand the role of the nurse. We have, in recent years, shifted things yet one more time, adding in the clinical nurse leader (CNL)[1] and doctor of nursing practice (DNP) programs to confuse the public and other members of the health care team even more. I am not saying that there is no value in these roles; quite the contrary. Having written the first CNL program in the New York City area, I am without a doubt committed to anything that will help enhance the quality of health care rendered to all. I see nursing leadership as integral to meeting this goal, and the creation of the CNL role is an intervention that has enormous potential to help fix significant issues in health care.

Some might ask why the CNL is considered an intervention with the potential to transform health care; a relevant question, but one that to me has an obvious answer and is germane to many of the topics discussed in this book. It is because the CNL student is being educated based on the core values and excellences of the nursing profession with a unique skill set.

The CNL student is being taught all about quality, safety, change agency, advocacy and assertiveness, professional quality of life and organizational behavior, ethics, and in the program I created, end-of-life care too. The CNL student is learning many of the foundational elements that have been downsized, or, on occasion, completely omitted in the nurse's primary or basic education. As a result, the CNL will be there to support and appreciate the carers—the bedside nurses and all the other staff who are so vitally important to the provision of quality caring. The CNL will be uniquely positioned to facilitate the enhancement of quality caring at the bedside. However, even with adequate education, staff nurses and CNLs cannot transform health care alone. We need staff nurses, administrators, educators, and APNs to have the same foundational elements in their education. The roles may differ, and with it the level of education, but the foundation should be the same.

Advanced practice nursing roles are of equal importance in our health care system and I certainly support pushing their education level up to a clinical doctorate (the DNP). The intricacy of multiple diagnoses and treatments, along with the chaos and complexity of the systems themselves, is such that more education is necessary to prepare APNs. Still, there remains the fact that we have had the clinical nurse specialist (CNS) role, which has never been clearly delineated. Having worked as a CNS, I can say that far too often CNSs find themselves in positions where they are not valued and where they have to repeatedly explain what they do and how it impacts on care outcomes as well as patient and staff satisfaction.

We have had the NP role, where NPs frequently work in a medical model and feel, for whatever reason, constrained by the organizational policies, which many times conflict with nursing's core values. All of these factor into the manifestation of burnout syndrome. So, the DNP is very important but will only be truly transformational if the educational programs that are being created include the teaching of all the things necessary to enhance knowing participation in change in addition to primary care expertise and clinical skills.

DNP programs need to include leadership, assertiveness and advocacy training, ethics, organizational behavior, and self-care—professional quality of life issues. End of life care education should also be included (at a minimum, full End of Life Nursing Education Consortium [ELNEC] training), and I say this not only because it is my preference, but because it is an area of unprecedented need in our society (and globally, for that matter). That some of my own colleagues in academia cannot see this is so very discouraging (see Chapter 9 for further discussion on this topic).

Educators should not assume that nurses coming into graduate programs already have any of this skill set, for it is likely that many do not. To be blunt, without all of it, APNs will continue to move along as they have in the past. Some will be much more effective than others; however, with the DNP *and* the skill set that includes learning how important nurses are and how to make our voices heard, the profession of nursing might finally move forward into the driver's seat where it belongs.

Minimizing what we refer to as the "art" of nursing—devaluing the importance of the compassionate caring practices of our work—along with the nondevelopment of advocacy and assertiveness skills has contributed to us having a workforce that has been relatively easy to oppress. Increasing our scientific knowledge while minimizing the study and application of the things that enable us to engage in caring practices has *not* empowered us. Instead, a vicious cycle has ensued—where the oppressed have become the oppressors, and this, in turn, has made many of our workplaces toxic, with bullying behavior rampant. All of these things contribute to stacking the deck.

The devaluing of the caring aspects of nursing includes the widespread teaching of depersonalization. Since burnout, at least in part, seems to stem from our inability to fulfill our inherent need to connect with others and to know that we are making a difference in the world, it does not make any sense to teach depersonalization. I have heard thousands of nurses and nursing students over the years say that they were taught *not* to use first names, *not* to cry in a patient's room, *not* to hug or show patients or their loved ones affection, *not* to become "emotionally" connected. Never were they taught how to just be present. Indeed, I too was taught in this manner. It is typically called "therapeutic use of self," and some semblance of this idea is taught in every health care profession. But it really is not therapeutic; it actually encourages the use of distancing when performing patient care. Pettigrew (1990) pointed out that therapeutic use of self is not the same as providing presence. He noted that a "nurse may be physically present, even attentive, and still refuse to give self in an interaction," whereas "presence . . . means making room internally for the other person, being willing to be involved, to be there wholeheartedly" (p. 503).

In the burnout literature, depersonalization is equated with cynicism and detachment from the job. And here we are, from the beginning, teaching our nurses that they need to maintain distance in order to do the job well. Some start off their careers already burned out! Or, at the very least, they become compassion fatigued early on, perhaps even while still in school. I have heard it said that we go into the profession of nursing with a naïve idealism that is quickly knocked out of us in the harshness of the workplace and that it is the real conflicting with the ideal that makes us more vulnerable to the syndrome of burnout. The fact is that naiveté alone cannot account for our vulnerability to burnout; *we* have to take responsibility for at least some of what ensues to ultimately "set us up" for these syndromes.

PHASES OF BURNOUT

Psychologists Herbert Freudenberger and Gail North (Kraft, 2006) identified a number of phases of burnout. They may not occur in any particular order, and they all do not have to manifest in order for someone to be experiencing burnout:

1. The Compulsion to Prove Oneself

2. Working Harder

3. Neglecting Their Needs

4. Displacement of Conflicts

5. Revision of Values

6. Denial of Emerging Problems

7. Withdrawal

8. Obvious Behavioral Changes

9. Depersonalization

10. Inner Emptiness

11. Depression

12. Burnout Syndrome (Kraft, 2006, p. 31)

Individuals who are developing burnout will frequently appear to be ambitious. Wanting to prove themselves, they work harder and harder, and as they try to demonstrate worthiness, they let go of other important things (Freudenberger & North, 1985), such as not taking care of themselves (eating and sleeping poorly) and spending less time with loved ones. It seems as if their values have changed—things that were important to them before no longer seem so.

At some point burned-out individuals become aware that there is something wrong, but they are unable to define it—it is at this stage that physical manifestations commonly begin to appear (Freudenberger & North, 1985; Kraft, 2006). Despite the recognition that something is wrong, many individuals will not confront the issues and instead become intolerant, cynical, and even aggressive (bullying behaviors may arise). Withdrawal, apathy, and depersonalization are characteristic and can lead to depression, with increasing feelings of hopelessness. At its most extreme, burnout syndrome can lead a person who is afflicted to thoughts of suicide and, for some, to eventual suicidal acts (Freudenberger & North, 1985).

So How Do You Know if You are Burned Out?

Exhaustion is said to be the classic sign of burnout; however, as a standalone, it does not capture the essence of this complex phenomenon, especially since compassion-fatigued individuals are also often exhausted physically, psychologically, and/or spiritually. Maslach (1993) identified three core dimensions of burnout: (1) an overwhelming feeling of exhaustion, (2) feelings of cynicism and detachment from the job, and (3) a sense of ineffectiveness and lack of accomplishment. Research in the area of burnout has led to the creation of various assessment tools, the predominant one being the Maslach Burnout Inventory (MBI), which measures all three dimensions (Maslach, Jackson, & Leiter, 1997).

Accumulating data suggest that there is a progression from exhaustion to cynicism over time, however, it remains unclear as to when feelings of ineffectiveness may come into play (Maslach, Schaufeli, & Leiter, 2001). Although the first and last dimensions are self-explanatory, the second—cynicism—requires an explanation. Many people take cynicism to mean sarcasm scorn and/or skepticism; however, as a dimension of burnout, cynicism really refers to feelings of pessimism, which then manifest as detachment and disengagement. As Leiter and Maslach (2009) noted:

> Burnout is one end of a continuum in the relationship people establish with their jobs, and stands in contrast to the opposite pole of engagement, in which people experience energy, involvement with their work, and feelings of effectiveness. (p. 332)

Thus, what we have is this:

Burnout	*Contentment*
Exhaustion	Increased energy
Disengagement ← ----------------------- → Engagement	
Feelings of ineffectiveness	Feelings of effectiveness

Unlike compassion fatigue, which is sudden in onset, burnout sneaks up on you, developing gradually over time. *Pfifferling* and *Gilley* (2000) differentiate between burnout and compassion fatigue by noting that individuals suffering from burnout tend to emotionally withdraw and display diminished empathy, whereas individuals with compassion fatigue will continue to give of themselves despite it wearing them down. It is said that if compassion fatigue is recognized and addressed early enough, burnout, which is more pervasive and difficult to recover from, may be prevented (Benson & Magraith, 2005).

Chenevert (1985) noted the importance of anger, how it helps us cleanse our minds and can also help renew our interest and enthusiasm for work. She also made the astute observation that anger may well be a precursor of burnout, noting that "usually before you burn out, you have to burn up" (p. 47). Herein one can see a clear relation to the topic of moral distress discussed earlier. The morally distressed nurse will feel frustration and anger; channeled appropriately, it can lead to butterfly power of a good sort. Anger is a meaningful transformation of energy; whether it is turned inward or outward, it is very meaningful. It means that change is needed. Just as a little bit of anxiety can be a good thing, a little bit of righteous anger can impel us to seek change, and that is always a good thing when you are unhappy with a set of circumstances. What we do not want is for moral residue to build up.

It has been noted that both compassion fatigue and burnout seem to arise as a result of failed survival strategies related to the inability to achieve one's goals (Valent, 2002). It would seem that burnout is a kind of defense mechanism similar to pulling your hand away from something hot. Shut the switch, pull the plug, become numb, and protect yourself. The difference and the irony is that in flicking the shut off switch, we actually hurt ourselves as well as others.

There are a great many signs and symptoms that may manifest when one is suffering from burnout. I especially like Chenevert's (1985) list, which includes whining and bitching, among other appropriately labeled common behavior patterns (p. 47). Typical signs and symptoms of burnout include physical and emotional exhaustion, feelings of hopelessness and/or helplessness, depersonalization-dehumanization, disenchantment, forgetfulness, apathy, irritability, melancholy, reduced efficiency, and discontent with achievement (Langle, 2003; Pross, 2006). Tack on all of the previously listed signs and symptoms of compassion fatigue noted in Chapter 6 that are not listed here and add in just about any other human indication of suffering (physical, psychological, and spiritual), and you have a pretty good picture of the enormity of the situation. Burnout is serious stuff.

The one thing that is absolutely a sure sign of burnout is when you *really* hate getting up and going to work. At that point you are in genuine trouble, and, unfortunately, so are your coworkers, your patients, and your loved ones!

To recap, compare, and contrast, the nurse who is *heartful* is manifesting love and caring; she will be a compassionate carer and in return will feel good. She still works terribly hard and rarely takes a break but does not feel fatigued at the end of the day; instead she feels energized and goes home thinking that her job has been done well. The meaning and purpose of her work are evident, from which comes a sense of contentment. Some would say she is in flow; others might call it second wind. It is all about energy transformation. This goes back to the earlier discussion on how we actualize our potentials. Conversely, the nurse who is *heart empty*, or seemingly *heartless*, is just the opposite; she is manifesting apathy and perhaps lethargy; she will be a dispassionate carer and will not feel good about herself. She feels exhausted, energy depleted, and never goes home feeling like her job has been done well. She feels disheartened, hopeless, joyless, and numb.

WHERE WAS THE NURSE?

Recently, an article came across my desk that focused on the care of "cancer survivors," prompting me to relive yet again my experience as a patient who had just had major surgery for uterine cancer. At the memory, I hemmed and hawed whether I should include this particular story here and finally my emotion won out. What follows highlights an especially horrid experience for me (Todaro-Franceschi, 2007).

I requested to have a private room postoperatively, but there were none. My roommate was very confused; she kept running over to my bed. At one point she wanted to smoke one of my mouth swabs. It was a neurological oncology unit and while it was not surprising to find confused patients there, I was a fresh post-op *total abdominal hysterectomy, bilateral salpingo-oophorectomy* (TAH BSO) with *lymphadenectomy patient* (with a suture line even longer than the name of the procedure), and I was fully cognizant although not very mobile. Needless to say, I was scared to death! I could not guard myself; it was difficult enough just to take deep breaths.

My family, having stayed until I was admitted to a unit, formed a body shield around my bed and was insistent that I be moved to a safer place. Where was the nurse who admitted me into this bed on this unit, I wondered? I recalled that as a staff nurse I had always tried to have final say as to which room on the unit my patients would be admitted. I know I would not have willingly put a fresh post-op patient in with a confused ambulatory patient.

After what seemed like an eternity, but I am sure was no more than an hour or so, I was moved into another room via bed with all the typical amount of banging into doorways and things along the way. The jarring added salt to the wound; my body already felt so badly beaten. My new room was empty, but there was room for two patients, and shortly afterward, someone was admitted into the other bed. The standard process of admitting histories, assessments, and treatments transpired. The physicians (there were two) were fairly loud and I lay there wondering, where was the nurse? The compassionate person who advocates for patients, the person who would diplomatically tell the physicians to take their discussion of their private lives outside?

After some time contemplating the idiosyncrasies of just trying to close my eyes in this unrelentingly noisy environment, I decided to try to advocate for myself. I spent some time wondering just how I should approach this. Should I tell the physicians to stop discussing their vacations while working with a patient? Should I tell them I am having difficulty getting comfortable and really need to try to sleep? Or should I quietly call the nurse and ask her to advocate for me? Finally, I just decided to use the call bell and asked the nurse if there might be an alternative place for me.

Another period of time went by. I was told that there (miraculously) was a private room and once again I was hauled via bed out of the room; of course, did you doubt? The bed banging into the doorway and down the hall, and I was unceremoniously dumped, or at least it felt so, into a private room, but I was so very relieved. For the rest of the evening and night until 8:00 the following morning, no one came to check my vital signs or to see how I was doing. It was ok, my husband and daughter were nearby, but still I could not help wondering, where was the nurse?

There was this doctor of osteopathic medicine (DO) specializing in gynecologic oncology who was covering for my surgeon and who came around every once in awhile, beginning on post-op day 1. She always started her assessment by saying, "my hands are cold," immediately before she put them on me to assess my wounded, distended, hurting abdomen. Her hands were like ice, though they did not really bother me since I was in nonstop hot flash mode, but still I wondered, why could she not rub them together and warm them up prior to touching her patients? In this instance I was a patient, not a nurse, and I thought that it was not my place to tell her how to handle her patients. But I know that as a nurse, had I noticed this DO's problem with cold hands, and had she tried to touch my patients after announcing repeatedly that her hands were cold, I would certainly have mentioned to her how quickly and easily she could warm her hands prior to laying them on *my* patients. I reflected that perhaps no one else had yet noticed this little problem.

The second night postoperatively I developed acute abdominal distention. In the middle of the night I started to have dry heaves; I hadn't eaten anything. My abdomen was huge and board-like. I called the nurse and she answered via intercom; I explained to her, in between these awful dry heaves, how I felt. She did not come to the room and instead proceeded to tell me via intercom that she would inform the doctor on call. I thought, if only I had a stethoscope. Then again, I knew there would be no bowel sounds. Not one nurse had touched my abdomen or listened for bowel sounds since I had been admitted to the unit. I rationalized this by reminding myself that it was a neurological oncology unit, though assessing bowel sounds is very basic nursing.

A little time went by, actually 45 minutes, but it felt like forever to me. I called the nurse again and this time she informed me via intercom that the physician was up on another unit taking care of a patient. I told her I really needed someone to come see me. A little while later she came in with an oral dose of the antiemetic zofran and proceeded to tell me the doctor "ordered" this for my abdominal discomfort, but that the doctor could not come to the unit to see me because she was making rounds on patients upstairs.

In between dry heaves, I tried to explain that I did not have any nausea. I pointed to my huge abdomen. Yet, she did not seem to understand or recognize the potentially serious nature of what was going on with me. She instead informed me that "there are some really sick patients on this unit" and that "it's already almost 5 a.m.; the doctor will be making rounds in an hour or so." Essentially, she implied that I could wait and finished with, "here is the medication, this is what the doctor 'ordered' for you." She put the medication on the bedside table and left the room.

At that point I was desperate, knowing well that the zofran would not help me one bit. How could it? But I took it anyway and proceeded to vomit the pill back out with my next dry heave. As I stared at the whole pill there in my emesis basin, my tears flowed, and I put the call bell on again. This time when the nurse answered through the intercom, I insisted that someone either get a physician immediately or provide me with my surgeon's home telephone number. Another period of time went by, and finally someone came to see me. It was the DO with the very cold hands.

For three days and nights postoperatively, I cared for myself with the help of my loved ones. After I received several laxatives, I could finally pass gas and no longer had dry heaves, but then I could not eat anything without having to go to the bathroom. And with the abdominal suture line the bedpan was even less friendly than it would usually be, and my sense of urgency was such that I was sure I would not be able to move quickly enough to get to the bathroom. So, I asked for a commode and one was brought into the room.

Since I had been admitted to this unit, no one had asked if I need anything, offered to assist me with bathing or to get out of bed and walk. I did my own I & Os and assessment. Not one person ever looked into the commode or offered to clean it out. Thank heaven for my family; they rotated shifts to be with me throughout this ordeal. My spirit was truly broken; I just could not imagine caring for anyone like this. I wondered if it was because I was not a neurological cancer patient, or because I was 47 and not elderly or younger, or because perhaps I had upset the nurses with my repeated requests for a private room.

An APN who covered this unit stopped in to visit. She was lovely, compassionate, and efficient. She asked me about everything and I told her a bit of my plight; my intestinal problems were consuming me still and she empathized with me. She told me that the unit is run mostly by travel nurses because there was a very high, frequent turnover of staff and that it was a hard unit for everyone to work on. I told her I understood how difficult the work of the nurse is, and that I was a nurse myself, but in my head I was thinking that having a *hard* job could not account for the dispassionate and sometimes substandard care I received during my stay there.

Four days postoperatively, still suffering with too frequent bouts of diarrhea, my daughter noted that there was no running water in the bathroom. I called the nurse and was told that they were doing renovations on another floor and she guessed that they had to shut off the water. I was told to be patient, but in the meantime, my loved ones could carry the dirty pot from the commode across the entire unit to the soiled utility room where they could rinse it. They could also get water from there and carry it back to my room. I was horrified.

Several hours into the day with no water, and several bowel movements later, my surgeon walked in on rounds with his entourage of staff. I broke down completely and in a fit of absolute despair and anger, I told him about my experience on this unit. I told him about his DO's cold hands, and about not being sick enough to warrant a nurse walking into the room or to have a physician come down to the unit to see me in the middle of the night when I was having such difficulty. I tried to explain what it felt like to have dry heaves 24 hours postoperatively with my abdominal suture line, and what it felt like to watch my loved ones, with no sleep, provide the care that I would willingly give to anyone as a nurse if he or she were my patient. What it felt like to be the recipient of such awful care, having been a nurse for over two decades and having dedicated my life to advocating and caring for people, both patients and nurses alike.

I told him that I could have been anything, could have done anything, but that I chose nursing because I love what I do; I love making a difference in people's lives. I told him how I have looked forward to getting up each morning and going to work, and that the few times during my career where I did not, I knew that it was time to change jobs and I did so. I pointed out that there were way too many folks at his hospital who obviously did not like getting up and coming to work each day.

I finished my heartfelt tirade with the fact that I had no running water in the bathroom for much of the day, that I had had too many bowel movements to count, and that my family was running back and forth across the unit to go to the soiled utility room to clean out the commode and to get water. He and his group of interns, residents, and an APN were very close to tears by the time I finished. It was clear that they were all appalled.

Truth be told, so was I. I had never intended "to wash my dirty laundry in public," so to speak. I was ashamed, for me and also for my profession.

Shortly thereafter, my surgeon had me transferred up to the gynecologic oncology unit. The minute I was wheeled onto the unit I felt the change in environment. It was far less stressed, the walls were painted in pastel colors, and there were motivational pictures all around. The nurses seemed so much happier, too. I felt better just being there, and while I had intuitively understood before, I now understand firsthand why Nightingale underscored the importance of the environment for healing. I felt an immense relief immediately upon arriving on that unit.

The following afternoon I was discharged from the hospital. What did I learn from this experience? I learned that the environment can make all the difference when it comes to healing and that it absolutely is not enough to have the best surgeon; one has to have compassionate, competent nurses to assist in the healing process. I experienced firsthand that disenchantment and dispassionate care go together and comprise key manifestations of the "ugly." The nurses who worked on the neurological unit were clearly unhappy, and it showed in the way they provided care for me. It almost seemed as if the nurse had disappeared entirely, and in her place was an unthinking, uncaring—inhuman—thing. A robot.

THE CONSEQUENCES OF BURNOUT

At this point, no one has to tell you what is at stake; still, I would like to stress that all of what is at risk begins with *our* own health and well-being. Very often the professional literature available to nurses—staff, leaders, and educators—focuses on issues of care-performance, quality, safety, productivity, outcomes, and so forth. Yes, that is all important and it is all one; however, at its center is *us*. We are the most important piece of the health care system. In fact, as I have already noted elsewhere (and will continue to do), we are so darn important that without *us*, the health care system will cease to exist. We must care for ourselves before we can be in an optimal place to care for others. We need to tend to us, personally, professionally, and wholly.

As previously noted, the refined model for Magnet hospitals includes five key components: transformational leadership, structural empowerment, exemplary professional nursing practice, new knowledge, innovations and improvements, and empirical outcomes (Wolf, Triolo, Reid-Ponte, Drenkard, & Moran, 2011). Notably, the model emphasizes the importance of the relational aspects of the work environment in a number of ways. Both patient and nursing satisfaction are given equal attention in addition to clinical outcome measures. The message is clear. It is just not enough to aspire to have great clinical outcomes; people satisfaction (people being both the cared for and the carers) is important too, and without addressing this, we may not be able to attain positive outcomes at all.

Economically, it is not savy to ignore the needs of the carers, especially nurse carers. By 2025, there will be an increased demand for, and reduced supply of, nurses, which will result in a shortage of 500,000 registered nurses (Buerhaus, 2008). We know that job satisfaction is the biggest predictor of whether or not one will stay in a position (Böckerman & Ilmakunnas, 2008), and while we often may not know which comes first, the dissatisfaction or the burnout, we do know that they are linked to one another (Maslach et al., 2001).

Replacing just one unhappy nurse who leaves her job can cost an organization up to $88,000 (and this figure is likely more by the time you read this). And unhappy nurses who stay on the job probably cost their workplaces even more. Absenteeism, lateness, and poor job performance/productivity are all associated with burnout, not to mention that a lack of commitment to the workplace results in a domino effect: it is contagious. So here we have just a few miserable burnt-out nurses on a unit; they call in sick, show up late, do not do their jobs well, and they are not nice to their coworkers. What happens? Everyone on the unit is affected, and ultimately the domino effect results in an ugly transformation of the quality of care rendered to people, people who are depending on and trusting us to care for them.

In one Canadian study, it was found that medication errors were linked to inadequate staffing and resources, feelings of exhaustion or overload, working overtime, poor nurse–physician relations, low coworker support, and low job security (Wilkins & Shields, 2008). All things that contribute to burnout. The dynamics of the whole must be acknowledged.

Complaisance Does Not Fit With Compassionate Care

A colleague of mine often talks about the power of a warm blanket. I would like to talk about the power of a pillow and the suffering that was caused by the complaisance of staff who had apparently become accustomed to not having adequate resources.

> *Having had major surgery for a life-threatening situation, the patient remained intubated the first night post-operatively. On extubation the next morning, his wife was allowed by his bedside for just a few minutes. The first words he said to his wife were, "What is behind my head?" But she could not get near him to examine it closely because of all the equipment in the room, although she could see that there was no pillow; instead there was a folded sheet beneath his head. At that moment the nurse manager walked in, and after speaking*

briefly to the patient—asking him how his pain was—she turned to the wife and told her that she had to leave immediately. Visiting hours started at 11 a.m., the wife was told.

As the wife left she asked his primary nurse to please get him a pillow and also check the back of his head. The nurse replied that they did not have any pillows on the unit but that they could try to "steal" one from another area. At 11 a.m., when the wife went back to her husband's bedside, he again complained of pain in the back of his head. Several chest tubes; multiple arterial, central and peripheral lines; a cracked chest, and all he was complaining about was the back of his head. On investigation, his wife found a large stage 3 bed sore across the entire occipital area; she was mortified, enraged, and felt guilty that she had ever let the nurse manager make her leave his bedside to begin with. He now had a pillow, but the damage was already done.

Working with inadequate resources or in an unhealthy environment, and having an administration that does not hear the voice of nurses when we assert ourselves on behalf of our patients, can result in complaisance. It should not happen, but it does. Due to the passivity (complaisance) of the staff, having gotten used to a lack of resources, this patient suffered with a draining and painful stage 3 bed sore during his recovery that persisted for months after discharge, along with occipital nerve damage, causing lasting numbing and painful headaches. It should not have happened, but it did.

Complaisance is one form of silence. Being acquiescent, not speaking up about things that affect your practice, for example, consistently working with a lack of basic resources, is passive unhealthy behavior. It is injurious because being silent about things that should matter leads to moral distress, moral residue, and, eventually, burnout. When a nurse is burned out, the apathy results in silence. Remaining silent about one's unhappiness extends to being silent about practice issues—issues the nurse no longer seems to care about. This can include bearing witness to all kinds of negative influences—both covert and overt. The burnt out nurse becomes a "silent voice" and a "silent witness."

APPLYING ART FOR HEALING BURNOUT

Remember when you first went into nursing? More than likely you were excited at the thought that you would make a difference in the lives of those you cared for. You looked forward to contributing to human health and healing and to learning the "how to's" of nursing. This was not because the things you learned were at the heart of nursing, but because learning the "how to's" got you closer to the essence of nursing: to care for, to assist with healing. Are you still eager? Recall the nurse who shared how she had changed from being outgoing and sociable while working with her patients to preferring to float to the emergency department where she could just "do her work" and not have to spend time interacting with her patients. Do you feel similarly disenchanted?

Step 1: Acknowledge a Feeling or Wound That Needs Healing

The first question you need to ask yourself (or if you are a nurse leader or educator ask your staff or students) is the one I offered at the beginning of the book. Do you look forward to going to work? If the answer is no, then you must ask why.

Are you working with people who do nothing but complain and who seem cynical, complaisant, and perhaps callous? Are you one of those people? Do you work with patients who are suffering and no longer feel any anguish on their behalf? Do you walk into a room with loved ones surrounding the bed of one of your acutely ill patients and shut a switch or block any exchange of feelings with your methodical actions to provide care?

As you go about your work, make an effort to be mindfully aware of the things that you dislike or things that you *used* to dislike and no longer notice. You may be surprised to find that there is a lot that used to bother you and no longer does. Such is the case with burned out carers. At some point, you will want to recapture those feelings related to the things that used to bother you. You want to acknowledge them because they hold the key not only to healing but also to evading compassion fatigue and burnout in the future. It might be helpful to draw two columns and label them as follows:

Reasons Why I Do Not Want to Go to Work	Reasons Why I Go to Work
1._____	1._____
2._____	2._____
3._____	3._____
4._____	4_____

Warning! If you are really unhappy, you might need more room for that column on the left, and if that is the case, take out your notebook or journal. You might also want to pick up the newspaper to begin looking for a new position!

Complete the burnout part of the questionnaire in Stamm's (2010) ProQOL survey in Appendix A. Are you manifesting any of the negative behaviors, feelings, and physical ailments related to burnout? Carefully reflect upon the reasons why you do not want to go to work. What seem to be the most outstanding things on your list? What is the deal breaker for you … is it your relationship with coworkers or other members on the health care team, workload, a lack of resources, or perhaps even the patient population you are working with? It could be anything—it is your responsibility to identify and acknowledge it. Once you do, you are ready to proceed to the next step. Since burnout develops over time and there are usually a lot of things contributing to it, your healing from it will not happen overnight. Be kind and patient with yourself.

Step 2: Recognize Choices and Take Purposeful Action

Once you have identified the reasons why you (or your staff or students) do not want to go to work, you are ready to explore how you might be able to change or facilitate changes in your workplace to enable you (or staff/students) to reaffirm purpose in your work. Are the reasons relational? In other words, is your unhappiness predominantly due to relationships with your leaders, coworkers, or others? Are you lacking a sense of communality—connectedness? Or is it related more to the physical environment?

Things such as chronic short staffing, high acuity, lack of resources such as linens, medications, and so forth, all make for a crummy physical environment, but there are other things that can contribute to an unhealthy workplace. A case in point was a story I heard at a conference several years back about a pediatric emergency room where there was no quiet place for families to go and be with their loved ones when a child died. The staff nurses were unhappy, to say the least. One day they got a great idea. There was a little closet off to the side, not much used. They asked for and received administrative permission to move everything out and went on to create a beautiful quiet space. It made a world of difference to the staff to be able to do that for those grieving families and alleviated a lot of additional suffering. Imagine the difference it made for the loved ones of the children who died.

Do you have things on your unit that are making you dislike your work? Can you make changes in your practice or the work environment that can help you to reaffirm your purpose? What choices do you have that might make things better for you and for your patients? List them. Can you approach your administrative staff alone or do you need the support of coworkers? Who might listen to your concerns and support you in making the necessary changes in practice?

Are you suffering with physical or mental health issues as a consequence of your work? If so, you need to make choices that will help you to regain your well-being. A first step is to meet with your primary care provider and talk about it. If you are feeling depressed or are self-medicating with food, alcohol, pills, or some other form of drug, now is the time to seek appropriate help for it. Remember, as knowing participants there are always choices we can make.

With burnout, it is important to recognize that even though you do have many choices, you may not be able to make things better enough to be able to stay in the work environment you are in and be happy or healthy. It may be impossible to regain your well-being and a sense of purpose working in the same place. It might be time for you to change positions. Some things can be fixed and some cannot. It is not a failure to acknowledge it is time to move on—it is a choice—and it may be the best one for you.

Step 3: Turn Outward Toward Self and Others

In order to heal from burnout once you have identified it, you must make a real effort to be mindfully aware of how you are acting and how others are acting in the workplace. In the literature on relational practices in organizations and systems, when important things like compassion and connection are overlooked, it is frequently referred to as "disappeared," because these important things are not "celebrated, valued or reinforced in any systematic way" (Frost, 1999, p. 130). To undo the harm of longstanding toxicity, we need to make these important things *reappear*. The way to do that is by turning outward—being mindfully aware that this is a process of relearning ourselves by noting patterns of negativity and replacing those patterns with attentive listening and presencing for both ourselves and others.

Reconnecting with our spiritual selves and perhaps one's religiosity is helpful, not only for finding meaning and purpose in life but in the seeming absence of it; our awareness of the interrelatedness of everything can help us to *make* meaning in our lives. Look for things you do not normally notice (or no longer notice). Remember the reconnect contention!

Prevention: "Burnin" and Brightly Burning

Prevention strategies for us as a profession need to begin in nursing education and then continue in practice environments. In one article written on the topic, nurse Kathleen Magill (1982) outlined a process that she called *burnin* to help future nurses develop the necessary coping skills that would enable them to become effective change agents. Burnin includes learning self-care strategies as well as conflict resolution and assertiveness skills.

Magill (1982) also wrote about what she called "the brightly burning," those nurses who were, despite everything, able to cope with stress and avert burnout. She suggested that it would be in our best interests to study those brightly burning nurses to identify their strengths, support systems, and change agency abilities. She noted that, "Most agencies seem to have some professional nursing personnel who manage to humanize and upgrade professional nursing practice in spite of conditions that burn out many other nurses" (p. 20). She went on to note: "If we focus exclusively on the burnout phenomenon in our nursing research, we may unwittingly build in a self-fulfilling prophecy that suggests that nurses tend to burn out" (p. 20).

When working as an upper level manager, Magill (1982) performed an informal survey of nurses who she considered to be "burning brightly," and while it was a small study ($N = 35$), with an admittedly biased sample, the results were quite interesting. Strong professional self-image, commitment to patients, risk-taking ability, and change agency skills were all apparent and fostered work satisfaction for these nurses. All of these things enhance compassion contentment and are in line with findings from various Magnet studies (Drenkard et al., 2011).

Perhaps the most important prevention strategy is to always hold first and foremost a sense of the meaning and purpose of our nursing work as carers. That has to come from within, but with mindful awareness we can keep it front and center to guide us in our day-to-day practice.

KEY POINTS

- Burnout is a result of interacting in negative ways with one's work environment.
- Burnout in nurses is an ugly transformation in which compassionate care is often replaced with dispassionate care.
- Many things contribute to the development of nurse burnout, including unresolved compassion fatigue, build-up of moral residue, the way one has been educated (or lack thereof), devaluing the art of nursing (the caring aspects of nursing) while stressing the science, inequity in treatment, lack of respect, unrealistic expectations (related to heavy workload, lack of resources, etc.), incivility and bullying in the workplace, (and the list goes on and on and on . . .).
- Healing can occur with (1) recognition of the problem and attentive self-reflection upon turning points and experiences that have led up

to its development, (2) exploring the choices one has and then choosing purposeful actions to take in order to heal, and (3) a conscious effort to turn outward to reconnect with yourself and others.

- It may not be possible to continue to work in the same place and heal from burnout. It might be necessary to change positions or workplace, in order to achieve a state of well-being and to reaffirm purpose in your work life.

- Remaining in a job or workplace when one is burnt out without seeking help to heal from the syndrome does a serious disservice to everyone—yourself, those you care for, those you work with, your loved ones, and the profession, collectively.

- Prevention strategies include reminding ourselves of the importance, meaning, and purpose of our work.

ENDNOTE

1. CNL is a registered trade mark of the American Association of Colleges of Nursing who created this new nursing role—the first new role in nursing in close to 40 years.

Part IV

FACING DEATH

These special functionaries ... may not always feel prepared for the serious and difficult problems that they face in their daily work. As I see it, the problems are of two kinds: (1) those that confront each practitioner as an individual and (2) those that involve the collectivity of practitioners—whether they be the staff on a hospital ward, the members of a cancer research team, or the workers in a nursing home. Both types of problems have their origins in certain paradoxical characteristics of the work expected of persons in the health-sickness and helping occupations. There is the dilemma of coming to terms with the two somewhat conflicting goals of practice: (1) the maintenance of life as manifest in recovery-focused activity and (2) the relief of suffering through effective utilization of comfort measures and palliation. The work centers around choices. These choices involve keeping someone alive or letting him go, remaining objective and detached or becoming subjective and involved, encouraging independency or allowing dependency. Finally, in this work there is the high stress of being in constant or frequent contact with life-threatening disease and its psychosocial concomitants.
—JEANNE QUINT

Chapter 9

BEING PREPARED TO CARE
FOR THE DYING

> *... The practitioner cannot avoid a confrontation with death. He*
> *needs to face and come to terms with two realities: the anxiety*
> *associated with thoughts of his own forthcoming death and the*
> *tremendous power to influence other people's lives inherent in his*
> *own work. Stated somewhat differently, the practitioner who*
> *experiences the shadow of his own death learns to approach*
> *the choices and decisions affecting other people's lives with*
> *humility and with respect for the fragile and tragic nature of the*
> *human condition.*
> —JEANNE QUINT BENOLIEL

KEY TOPICS

- Death education and its importance for nurses
- Medical futility and moral distress

Nurses who regularly work with people who are dying know that there is always a last dose, a last meal, a last word, a last breath. Knowing that does not make it easier, especially when the loved ones are there bearing witness to the last everythings. Yet, there is something immensely sacrosanct about it. The memories of those last days will live forever in the hearts and minds of all those involved. Facing death with patients and their loved ones is an opportunity for us in nursing to make all the difference.

Although caring for dying patients and their loved ones offers us a chance to develop and provide sustaining memories at the most vulnerable times in people's lives, many nurses are not equipped with the necessary skills to deal with dying and death. I faced death on a regular basis when I was in nursing practice and, in retrospect, I can admit I was not always very good at it. Having never been educated in how to care for the dying, it was not something I thought much about when I entered into the profession, although soon enough I learned that it was going to be a part of my practice, whether or not I wanted it to be.

CODE 99, AGAIN?

I recall my first patient who died on a medical surgical unit; she was 93 years old, emaciated, and unresponsive, and we coded her, four times. I am certain ribs were cracked, and I distinctly remember my extreme worry when some of the interns and residents began talking about doing a "slow code" the next go-round if she was revived that last time. I was grateful that she did die and I did not have to witness or participate in any slow codes for her. Still, I did not sleep for days afterward. I just never thought anyone would die on my watch. I remember thinking, no one prepared me for this part of nursing. I was told that "slow codes" were illegal, for heaven's sake! I did not sign up to be a felon, did I?

I never thought kids die too ... But a year or so later, having been floated for the evening tour into the pediatric emergency room, I was forced to deal with the reality that no one is exempt from death. A 5-year-old with asthma coded, twice. She died a few weeks later in the pediatric intensive care unit (PICU), although technically she was considered "brain dead" after that first night. She was an only child in an Italian family, and the parents, grandparents, aunts, and uncles were present 24/7 at the hospital.

I was floated to the PICU twice during the time the child was on that unit and I remember staying clear of the visiting area where all of the family members were. I recollect being grateful that I only floated to these areas and did not have to work in them regularly. I also recall floating years later into the PICU at another hospital and being assigned to work with an 18-month-old in full-blown AIDS. I held him all night, both of us crying for much of it. Another time I floated to the neonatal intensive care unit (NICU) where there were so many babies teetering on the brink of death, and thankfully I was assigned to work with a preemie who suffered with sleep apnea. All I had to do during my time with him, aside from the normal bathing, feeding, and changing, was to flick the bottom of his foot with my finger every now and then to remind him to breathe. And breathe he did, at least for that shift. I do not know if he made it out of the NICU; when tours like that ended, I tended to book out of the hospital like my tail was on fire, without looking back lest something pull me back in there. You know how they say, do not take your work home with you? Those were the mornings when I was tempted to join coworkers as they pulled into the convenience store to buy their wine coolers or beer. I rarely did, but I was tempted, *a lot.*

As a cardiac clinical nurse specialist, I was once called upon to work with a woman with severe cardiomyopathy who had chosen to get pregnant despite the risk. Post-delivery she died and her newborn child lived. Going back to those idioms—do not take your work home with you, shut the switch, leave your work at work—well, that might be possible with papers, numbers, and other things. Rarely is it possible when you are dealing with human beings who are suffering and/or coworkers who are either suffering or, conversely, causing others to suffer. It is pretty hard to shake that kind of work off when you leave to go home at the end of the day, evening, or night.

No one ever talked about the possibility of these death experiences when I was a nursing student. We were taught Kubler-Ross's (1969) five stages of death in psychology, but that was really the extent of our education in this area. We were taught basic postmortem care—how to clean and wrap a body after death. We were never taught how to make eye contact with the patient who was dying, or his loved ones who asked, "Is he dying?" We were never taught how to talk, or listen, for that matter, to patients nearing the end of life. And we were certainly never taught how to comfort those who were left behind after their loved ones died.

Unfortunately, that still seems to be the norm in many schools of nursing; the emphasis is on health, and the prevention and cure of disease. Nowadays we emphasize healthy aging. It amazes me how we can focus on the maintenance and restoration of health, without acknowledging that, at some point, no matter what we have done or will do, death is going to occur.

TEACHING ABOUT DEATH

Since going into academia full time in 1997, I have made teaching about death, dying, and bereavement my main priority and focus for both teaching and scholarship. I have suffered the sometimes slow, and sometimes far too quick, inevitable death of dear loved ones, and I joined the prestigious group called "cancer survivors" in 2003. Up until then, I thought I knew everything one could know about dying and death; however, I found that dwelling with cancer on such a personal basis gave me an even more tangible sense of the fragility of life and living. In any case, I would say I am pretty well rounded with respect to end-of-life care issues.

Today, I am considered a "death educator," not in nursing but in my own transdisciplinary circle of thanatology scholars. Nursing, medicine, psychology, and social work have yet to embrace the idea of "death education," and this is really dismaying because death, like birth, is integral with health and healing. Indeed, many health care professionals believe that associating the terms *dying* and *death* with any kind of health care is destined to turn people away, rather than turn them toward seeking care. This is especially so with palliative care, where it is often erroneously believed that palliative care is something we only provide at the end of life. Thus, many of the folks working in palliative care make an effort not to talk about "end of life care" for fear it will taint the picture and prevent people from seeking care altogether.

What people fail to understand is that palliative care is holistic care aimed at preserving quality of life—and it need not be associated with dying and death. But, and this is a *big* but, at no other time is palliative care more fitting than when people are known to be approaching death. For it is when we acknowledge that we are approaching death and that life is indeed finite that many of us will value ever more readily what living is all about, and, thus, will want to be able to appreciate every single moment we have left. Palliative care is the means to that end.

I could fill another book with my experiences as an educator trying to teach this content over the years, and perhaps one day I will. But for now I will focus on the key points related to the topic at hand, which is our individual and collective professional quality of life. From my perspective, I see this as irrevocably connected with our ability to deal with death, to be able to face it—perhaps, on a daily basis—and work with it permeating our own lives, point blank, plain and simple.

As a nurse educator, it troubles me that we can expect nurses to work in all areas of health care with so many people and, yet, we continue *not* to prepare nurses to deal with dying and death, and loss in general. Repeatedly I hear from students who would be nurses that they do not *expect* to work with dying patients. I hear even more from nurses who come back to school for their BS or MS degrees that they were *never* taught how to work with dying patients and how uncomfortable they are doing so, and this is sometimes decades after they have been in practice! How unfair this is to them, the nurses, and how unfair it is to those who receive care *from* them.

My recent research exploring critical care nurses' perceptions of preparedness to care for the dying and its relationship to their professional quality of life gave me a huge amount of data that indicates there is a significant relationship (Todaro-Franceschi, unpublished data). Over 500 nurses from around the country participated in the study. The majority, when asked where they had learned to provide end-of-life care, answered "at the bedside." One nurse said, "I feel like I am in a chronic state of PTSD," and she probably is.

In my elective class, *Changing the Face of Death* (the class from which come most of the AHAs!), countless RN to BSN nurses pass through. Some enroll in the course just because it fits their schedule or they need an elective. More often, it is because they acknowledge a lack of preparedness to care for the dying. Other times, it is because they either are anticipating or have experienced the death of a loved one. It never ceases to amaze me how great the attendance is in this class, even when it is offered late in the evening. The student engagement is so palpable and I am always humbled by their stories and their AHAs. The following is one from an ED nurse.

> *Mid-December I found out that a dear colleague and friend whom I've worked beside in the ED and known for 4 years was diagnosed with end-stage pancreatic cancer. He was 50 years old. His name was Brian .... Brian taught me how to put a 14 Gauge in a critical patient, and was always the first to start ordering late night pasta deliveries for all of us stuck in the ED at 3am. He was a source of knowledge and laughter for us all. I attended to Brian's bedside several nights a week for about 5 weeks. He went home on hospice on Friday, January 22nd, led out of the ED from the ambulance bay with a standing ovation from all the ED staff and the EMS crews. It was a priceless moment I, and his family, will cherish forever.*
>
> *I spent the next few nights at Brian's home with his family and our other colleagues from the ED. We had hot tea in the snowstorm, we recanted humorous stories about him from triage, and we looked through his photo books with his Mom. On Wednesday, January 27, Brian was in respiratory distress and was breathing at approximately 50 respirations a minute. He was holding on and holding on, like he was scared to let go. Myself and three other nurses, along with his mom and dad, turned on some instrumental music I had on my iPhone, gathered round his bed, touched him, and I began to recite poetry and prayer. We all spoke to him and told him that it was OK to go. We gave him a dose of pain medication, and 8 minutes later he took his last breath.*
>
> *It was finally over. The streets were silent and covered with 2 feet of snow. Outside the midtown apartment in Manhattan, it was so peaceful. He chose the most beautiful night in New York City to die.*
>
> *My AHA moment was the very first class meeting when Dr. Todaro-Franceschi explained the purpose of this course and the mission of her teachings. I recall sitting in the back, on the highest row of chairs and I cried for the first time since I had found out Brian was ill. I had my moment because I realized that it is okay to grieve—even when you are a nurse in the ED. I am not just supposed to be a stone cold body expected to deal with it all as it comes at me.*

I can grieve as a friend, as a nurse, and as a person. I never realized why I hadn't shed a tear over Brian and that moment in class it all made sense.

I had been desensitized over the years I have been an ED Nurse. I had always practiced the art of "dealing with it and getting over it and moving on"—and fast. Get that body out of that room; I've got 30 patients waiting for a stretcher. My AHA was a special moment for me because I finally realized that not only am I an ED Nurse, but I am also an individual filled with emotion. Simply by me expressing that emotion does not take away from my Hard Core Emergency Room Edge and Attitude—it enlightens it.

It does not surprise me that the RN who shared her story had suppressed her feelings time and time again while working in the ED and facing death. Some might think, as she noted, that it is due to being desensitized over the years. It is more likely a combination of things that contributed to her behavior, and I am certain that part of it is the education (or lack thereof) that she received. If we are not taught how to face death during our education, most of us learn how to do it while working, at the bedside. That does not mean we learn how to do it well. For some, facing death means evading it, denying it, and fighting it. For some, it means not showing one's emotion, fragility, or humanness.

Occasionally I have had a hospice or palliative care nurse register for and attend my classes. More often than not, these nurses have such a good handle on caring for the dying that they become co-facilitators in our class discussions. These are also the nurses who seem less likely to burn out—they really love what they do. A recent review of the literature on the occurrence of burnout in palliative care indicates that there is *not* a higher incidence of burnout in this area of practice (Pereira, Fonseca, & Carvalho, 2011). In fact, some studies performed in the United Kingdom with physicians indicate that the incidence of burnout may be lower in palliative care than in other health care areas (Baumrucker, 2002). It makes enormous sense to me; these folks know how to face death, and because of it, they also know how to appreciate life.

What is clear is that working in hospice and palliative care settings is a choice that some nurses and physicians make; accordingly, these individuals make a point of developing the skills needed in this area of practice. That includes being able to connect with and talk to others about dying and death—communicating with the dying and their loved ones—as well as facing death on a regular basis.

Recently a student stopped me in the lobby of our campus building and asked if I had office hours. I did not know her, but I said sure, as I sat down next to her. She told me she was a senior in our generic program and that she had, along with another 125 students, recently attended two of the mandatory end-of-life care seminars I taught.

The student proceeded to tell me about a patient who had died during one of her clinical experiences:

> *The patient died right in front of me. She was a 70-year-old woman, who had been admitted some time before in heart failure with a bunch of other problems, including several infections that couldn't be controlled. She was unresponsive. I felt a bit anxious during the day; the woman was DNR and was desaturating as the day went on, but I continued to stay in the room and provide care for her. She started to have a change in her breathing, and then she died. I was upset and afterwards I cried even though I felt good that I was able to care for her. It was sad.*

> *When the staff saw me crying, they were cold and seemed so uncaring, but I was really upset by the instructor who said, "Why are you crying? You didn't know her; there is no need to cry." I was actually more upset about the reactions of the nurses and my instructor than the death of the patient.*

She told me that by the nurses and the instructor denying her the right to feel sad and to cry, she felt they were invalidating both the woman's life and her emotions.

As the student was telling me this story, she was visibly upset. She asked me if it was wrong for her have felt sad and to have cried the way she had. She said, "There was nothing I could do for this woman." To that I said, "It sounds like you did a lot. What did you do for her as she lay there in her final moments dying?" She responded, "I sat there beside her and held her hand," and with that, she burst into tears and, heck, so did I. My response to her was that there is nothing wrong with crying and showing human emotion. I told her that it is the nurse who *doesn't* cry that worries me.

Jean Quint Benoliel (Benoliel, 1973; Quint, 1967) documented the issues related to us caring for the dying patient—the need for better preparation in nursing education, both didactic and clinical—almost 50 years ago. Yet here we are still trying to deny its import—in both education and practice. It is time for us to take Jeanne Quint Benoliel's work to heart and get end-of-life care education to be mandatory and consistently taught in nursing programs. It is time to pull those MDs, social workers, psychologists, and chaplains into it, too.

DISTANCING AND DISCONNECTING:
DEATH DENYING PERSISTS

One would think that, by now, human beings would have come to terms with death and what has been referred to since the 1400s as the *ars moriendi*—the art of dying. Since ancient times, humans have philosophized and reflected upon dying and death. Yet, the thought of our death and that of loved ones evokes fear in most, if not all people, and consequently we choose not to think about it—not to go there. It is one of those places that really scare us.

We live in a death denying society and most nurses work in areas where we fight off death every day. However, there does come a point where fighting death will not prevent it from occurring. We know this but many still manage to bypass its reality, most of the time.

In her decisive work, *On Death and Dying*, Kubler-Ross (1969) noted that patients who are dying need to be afforded opportunities to share their concerns:

> ... It is evident that the terminally ill patient has very special needs which can be fulfilled if we take the time to sit and listen and find out what they are. The most important communication, perhaps, is the fact that we let him know that we are ready and willing to share some of his concerns. (p. 269)

Yet, what is the first thing many of us in health care do when we enter the room of someone who is dying? We blatantly ignore or try to deny the reality that death is at the door. Many refuse to talk about it with the patient or family, acting as if everything is normal. We maintain the status quo. In essence, most of us go about providing care, as if the patient is going to go home, resume previous activities, and live forever. Like Morrie said, in *Tuesdays with Morrie* (Albom, 1997), we fill the air, talking about things of little or no importance.

Over a decade ago, I wrote:

> Dying, for many, has become a cold, isolated process—cold in the sense that it is hard-core machinery touching the patient, rather than the gentle grasp of a familiar loving hand; isolated in the sense that strangers rather than family and friends often surround patients in their last living moments, strangers who are valiantly trying to prolong life .... It is the rare person who would consciously choose to die among strangers and yet in many areas of healthcare today we, in essence, force those who are dying to do so.
>
> —*Todaro-Franceschi, 1999, p. 130*

Have things changed much since then? I do not think so.

Surveys indicate that most people would prefer to die at home, however, less than a third of patients who are considered to be terminally ill enroll in hospice programs. Approximately half of the projected 2.5 million annual deaths in the United States take place in a hospital (Last Acts, 2002), and in most European countries, the majority of people continue to die in hospitals as well (Davies, 2004). Every year in the United States, over half a million people die in an ICU or after having had treatment while in an ICU during their last hospital admission (Angus, Banranto, & Linde-Zwirble, 2004).

Medically futile (or non-beneficial) treatment is becoming a mainstay, the outcome of which is tortuous death for many patients (Zhang et al., 2009). A recent report notes that approximately one third of Medicare patients with advanced cancer die in hospitals and ICUs and many of these patients are aggressively treated until they die (Goodman et al., 2010). Cap off this knowledge with the abysmal fact that one in four patients nearing the end of life continue to describe inadequate pain management and one in three families report that they receive insufficient emotional support (Center to Advance Palliative Care and the National Palliative Care Research Center, 2008), and we are indeed given a moral imperative to find a way to do things better.

When the Institute of Medicine (IOM) published a report in 1997 about end of life care, it became quite clear that there were deficiencies in all health care areas regarding dying and death. Further exploration in nursing by the American Association of Colleges in Nursing (AACN) led to a joint effort by AACN coupled with the City of Hope National Medical center (COH) to formulate the End of Life Nursing Education Consortium (ELNEC) to address the lack of end of life care curricular content in nursing education across the country (AACN & COH, 1999; COH & AACN, 2011). This effort, led by palliative care nurse pioneer Betty Ferrell, was initially funded by the Robert Wood Johnson Foundation in 1997 and continues today. In recent years it has expanded into an incredible global effort. Nursing is not alone in this endeavor; a similar effort has been made to address the end of life care deficiencies in medicine (Education in Palliative and End-of-Life Care [EPEC] project).

Despite the huge effort being made to rectify deficiencies in end of life care education for nurses, a recent study (Todaro-Franceschi & Lobelo, unpublished data), in which we surveyed nurse educators in schools of nursing around the country, indicates that there continue to be obstacles with getting end of life care content into nursing curricula. According to those who returned surveys ($N = 233$ completed the survey; participants represented all states with the exception of Alaska, Hawaii, Maryland, Utah, and Wyoming), the biggest obstacles appear to be faculty and administrative resistance. Even in schools where there are death educators, end of life care is not always being taught. Given the fact that it is, most of the time, us—the nurses—who are the strangers surrounding dying patients and their loved ones during their final days of life, it is up to us to help the transition from life to death, for both patients and their loved ones. Thus, the continued omission of death education in nursing is actually socially unjust for everyone (Todaro-Franceschi, 2011b, c).

Kubler-Ross (1969) wondered if our actions (our denial of death as carers) might really be defense mechanisms—our way of coping with and repressing the anxieties that an acutely or terminally ill patient evokes in us. She pointed out that the dying patient is suffering more today, not less, and asked, are we becoming more or less human? It does often seem that many who work in the various health care fields entirely forget that they are dealing with fellow human beings, not only those working in practice but also those in education teaching others to engage in practice. Take, for example, all the people going for these risky surgeries and procedures who are forced to spend days (and nights) beforehand, alone or with strangers who are poking and prodding them, rather than with loved ones during what might well be, and often enough turns out to be, their final hours.

In an exploratory study of seven individuals with advanced cancer, Coyle (2006) noted that it is hard work to *live* in the face of death. Ferrell and Coyle (2008) expand upon this in their book on suffering, emphasizing the fact that *working* in the face of death is also incredibly hard work; nurses have to be prepared to do it and to do it well.

A dear friend of mine, a perinatal clinical nurse specialist, used to care for women who were at high risk during their pregnancies. These were women who had gestational diabetes, hypertension, or HIV, among other things. Invariably (and far too often it seemed), the babies of some of her patients would die (*in utero* or immediately after birth). She would bathe and dress those babies and sit with the parents and loved ones, giving them time to grieve. I always said that if she did that once a year she would be earning her salary tenfold and that I could never do it. Her response to me was why ever not? She always believed it was a gift to be present during both birthing and dying; she said you cannot get closer to God then at those times. To embrace the living–dying process transforms us and those we care for. The rewards are life and death altering for everyone involved.

IS IT NECESSARY OR NOT?

Prolonging or sustaining life with little expectation that it will result in survival, or, if one does survive, a quality life, is considered medical futility. What is and is not considered medically futile care is a complex issue, and it is well-debated in the literature. Renowned bioethicist Dan Callahan

(1991) outlined the debate in his discussion of "the-problem-without-a-name," as he described what is considered medical necessity versus what is medically futile. How does one identify what is and is not necessary medical care?

Narrowed down to quantitative and qualitative roots, it has been noted that if a treatment is not expected to succeed, it is *quantitatively* futile, whereas if a treatment is expected to prolong life, but the quality of life is subsequently diminished, it is *qualitatively* futile (Schneiderman, Jecker, & Jonsen, 1990). Obviously this is problematic because none of us have a crystal ball that can predict for sure whether our actions will benefit or harm others. Thus, Schneiderman and colleagues advocated that we think in terms of probability. However, Callahan (1991) argued that this may well not be sufficient because, in health care, there is a distinct difference between how we approach the individual versus the collective.

What may likely be good for most is not necessarily good for all, and while we know this to be so, we still value "evidence-based practice" and emphasize predictability. However, evidence-based practice cannot assure an outcome will be what we want or expect it to be. Nurses who are at the bedside of critically ill patients know how suddenly a patient can turn around. Many oncology nurses will tell you that prognosis means little in the day-to-day scheme of things. It is all about the quality of living–dying. So how do we know we are doing the right thing? Can we ever know?

Before health care became so technologically savvy, people got acutely ill and died in a short space of time. Now we get acutely ill and die slowly over time. The entire problem of medical futility stems not just from technologic advances that can lead to cure, but societal expectations of those techno-cures. No one is talking about the risks associated with them. No one really says, well, at the age of 80, having surgery for some slow-growing cancer might kill you or result in a prolonged hospital stay with all kinds of nasty complications, whereas you could possibly live quite a while with cancer and have a great quality of life for much of that time. That is why, when the Patient Self-Determination Act came into being in the early 1990s, it was great in principle but failed in actuality. No one wants to have *the* talk.

Nurses are caring for people who are receiving non-beneficial care—this is traumatizing, in and of itself. In one survey of nurses across a wide range of settings including ER, ICU, hospice, and long-term care, significant moral distress was reported related to aggressive care and denying the need for palliative care (Ferrell, 2006). In critical care areas and emergency departments, many nurses are dealing with moral distress related to medical futility every single day, and some studies indicate that nurses working in these areas may be at increased risk for the development of both compassion fatigue and burnout (Hooper, Craig, Janvrin, Wetsel, & Reimels, 2010; Meltzer & Huckabay, 2004).

We recognize when care is most likely medically futile, but without adequate preparation during professional education, how can we advocate for these patients? Not having been taught how to communicate with patients and their loved ones about their living–dying choices, not knowing how to assert ourselves in order to make our voices heard, we wind up being a wounded workforce—morally distressed—all the while continuing to provide care that we know may not make much, if any, appreciable difference, and that may well be causing more harm than good.

My observations, both formal and informal, indicate that those who feel unprepared to care for the dying and their loved ones are at greater risk for compassion fatigue. Some of my research data also suggests that those who do feel well prepared to care for the dying may be at risk for burnout over time. Intuitively to me it makes sense, because the health care system as a whole does not acknowledge the acuity of the dying patient or the acuity of loved ones as recipients of care. Oh, we talk a good talk. Administration and those in charge may say that the family members are our patients too, but seldom, if ever, are they counted in acuity for staffing needs.

The patient whose life we are trying to save, even if futile, the one with all of the life-saving and life-preserving procedures, equipment, and medication, is a higher acuity than the patient who we have accepted to be in his or her final hours or days transitioning from life to death. In advanced labor and during delivery, a patient usually has a one-to-one carer; for people who are known to be dying, this is rarely the case. This logic has spilled over into our educational programs for nurses (and for physicians and other health care professionals). Or perhaps the logic we apply in practice stems from our education (or lack thereof). The question of which came first might be very relevant, but it is a topic for another time. The point is, rare is the nursing program that requires a full-term course on the topic, and, in fact, there sometimes seems to be a hidden curriculum in health care professional education that devalues the learning of thanatology topics entirely (Billings et al., 2010; Todaro-Franceschi, unpublished data).

WHY IS IT IMPORTANT FOR US TO BE PREPARED TO FACE DEATH?

After years of difficulty getting end of life care education to be a permanent fixture in the undergraduate program where I work, I set out to do an alumni study. I wanted to document what I intuited from both my practice and from my experiences teaching. The results of that study are reported in another publication, so I only offer a brief synopsis here (Todaro-Franceschi, 2011a, b). Students were surveyed to ascertain whether they perceived that the education they received at our school had adequately prepared them to care for the dying. They were also asked if they thought that their end of life care education has had an impact on their practice and their way of being in the world. "Changes in one's way of being in the world" was defined as an enhanced appreciation of people, places, and/or things; being more appreciative of life, generally speaking. Comparisons were sought between those who had taken the elective course and those who had not.

Findings revealed statistically significant differences among groups in their perceptions of preparedness to care for the dying as well as perceived changes in both practice and ways of being in the world (total $N = 154$ both generic and RN to BSN students), with those who had taken the elective reporting feeling better prepared and also more appreciative of life (Todaro-Franceschi, 2011a, b). A salient number of the RN participants who had chosen to take the elective offering in EOL care reported working in critical care (29%) and emergency departments (13%; over 42% of RN respondents), which suggests that nurses working in these areas feel more of a need to be prepared to face death. We should take note of the fact that accumulating research data on compassion fatigue and burnout in nursing suggests that in ED, intensive care, and oncology there is a high incidence of these syndromes. These are areas where nurses face death all the time.

Some folks, nurse faculty colleagues and students among them, have asked me over the years why I think it is so important for us to learn how to face death. The following is my answer:

- Because death is 100% guaranteed for every one of us.
- Because we ALL will have to face death, personally and professionally.
- Because doing it poorly hurts us.
- Because doing it well, while difficult, can infuse us with appreciation for life and living and help us live our moments joyfully and heartfully.
- Because our patients need us to help them face it.
- Because our patients' loved ones need us to help them through it.
- Because the cost of aggressive health care at the end of life is astronomical and does not usually result in enhancing the quality of living while dying.

APPLYING *ART* IN PREPARATION OF CARING FOR THE DYING

Coming to terms with the possibility that you (or your colleagues and staff) may have a problem with facing death and are ill-prepared to care for the dying is important—again, you cannot fix what you do not recognize or acknowledge as broken. There are many purposeful actions that can be taken to help one feel more prepared to care for the dying and their loved ones. We can become more comfortable with it, and although it will never be an easy thing to do, we can find meaning and purpose in the experiences we have with the dying. Of course, it is a choice you have to make. Some people cannot, or do not want, to face death at all, and that is ok. What is not ok is that we deny another's experience of it by flicking that shut off switch. If you are regularly facing death and decide that you do not want to deal with it, it will be far better for everyone if you go work in a different area entirely.

Step 1: Acknowledge a Feeling or Wound That Needs Healing

Ask yourself if you avoid speaking about dying and death with others, personally and professionally. Is the topic of death "taboo" in your culture? Generally speaking, do you feel able to provide quality care to the dying and their loved ones? You may wish to complete the questionnaire about perceptions of preparedness located in Appendix B of the book.

Sometimes our previous experiences with death "set us up" for how we act in similar situations. Realize that "similar" in this instance simply (or not so simply) means occurrences where dying and death happen—*dying (usually) leads to death*—all have that in common, although every single event of death is unique. You may have had personal or professional experiences that have set you up to be uncomfortable with dying and death. For instance, the student who shared with me how the staff and her instructor ridiculed her for crying and being sad—that might have discouraged her from sharing her feelings in the future, were it not for the fact that she chose to approach me to discuss what had happened. I am hopeful that she will remember my saying that it is the nurse who does not cry that worries me.

Do you ever cry for those who are dying or have died? Did you used to cry easily but no longer do? If you answer in the affirmative, it may be time to go back to Chapter 8 on burnout. Then again it might not; only you can assess whether or not you are distancing yourself from experiences that may be painful. Only you can say for sure if you are evading the places that scare you.

If you work in an area where patients frequently die, and your staff or coworkers seem to be uncaring or dispassionate, encourage them to explore their feelings regarding dying and death. A focused group discussion on the topic can be very useful to identify areas where more staff preparation may be needed.

Step 2: Recognize Choices and Take Purposeful Action

First, ask yourself if you want to learn to be more comfortable with dying and death. If so, please see the resource section on end of life care education. There are many courses available on the subject. If you are in the New York City area, stop in on one of mine! If you are not interested in becoming more comfortable with dying and death, it might be that you need to do some self-reflection related to experiences you may have had with dying, death, and bereavement. Once you have identified areas that may be contributing to your discomfort with dying and death, the following are some choices you might consider:

- Taking an ELNEC course (please see the resource section)
- Enrolling in a university course on dying and death (check your local college)
- Speaking with a spiritual advisor (e.g., your rabbi, priest, pastor, etc.)
- Speaking with friends and loved ones about it
- Doing some grief work with a counselor or support group

Depending upon your unique situation, there will be other choices and actions that you can think about. Once again, you may decide that facing death is not something you can do or want to do. If that is the case, list alternative choices and strategies such as changing your area of practice or even changing your nursing role entirely. What you must not do is continue to work in an area where you feel compelled to deny death, although you are forced to deal with it. This choice and concurrent action will lead to turning away from the problem—flicking that shutoff switch, which is unhealthy for you and definitely not helpful for others.

Step 3: Turn Outward Toward Self and Others

At no other time is it more imperative for us as carers to turn outward toward ourselves and others than when we face death. Of course, some of my colleagues say I am biased, since I am so passionate about death education. I do not think that is it at all. Turning outward toward ourselves and others is so important when facing death, because having an appreciation of ourselves and our connectedness to all else enables us to live more fully. Recognition that life is fleeting, and seeing, really seeing the things we take for granted every day can help make us feel *heartful*.

If we are able to face the fact that death happens to everyone and as a result can appreciate our moments as we live them, we will be in a better position to help those who are living their final days and moments. We will be more able to go to the places that scare us and them, *with* them.

Facing death with them, we bear witness to their suffering, and are able to put ourselves in the person's place because we understand that one day we and our loved ones will be in that same place. As Morrie said, "learn how to die, and you learn how to live" (Albom, 1997, p. 83). We have to be able to turn outward in order to appreciate living and dying. If we are *really* enjoying life, it is because we are turning outward toward ourselves and others, in most, if not all, of our moments. Morrie

> . . . nodded toward the window with the sunshine streaming in. [He said] "You see that? You can go out there, outside anytime. You can run up and down the block and go crazy. I can't do that. I can't go out. I can't run . . . But you know what? I *appreciate* that window more than you do . . .. I look out that window every day. I notice the change in the trees, how strong the wind is blowing. It's as if I can see time actually passing through that window. Because I know my time is almost done, I am drawn to nature like I am seeing it for the first time.
>
> *—Albom, 1997, p. 84*

Without self-reflection and forcing ourselves to face this most complex and, for many, terrifying subject, we never come to face the finite nature of life. We go through our days never realizing that this moment, this *right now*, is the only *right now*, and it may be the *last right now* there is for us, our loved ones, our patients, and their families.

KEY POINTS

- Death happens; its 100% guaranteed.
- Everyone is going to face death, whether prepared for it or not.
- Nurses who work in areas with people who are dying are especially vulnerable to compassion fatigue and moral distress because they are the ones at the bedside bearing witness to suffering, both from medically futile care and from the "failure to cure."
- Nurses need to learn how to be more comfortable facing death and to develop the concomitant skills necessary to care for the dying and their loved ones.
- Being unable to face death results in flicking the shutoff switch (denying and defying death), which is unhealthy for us and does a disservice to the patient who is dying and his or her loved ones.
- Learning how to face death can teach us how to appreciate life.

Chapter 10

SHARED HORRORS AND ACHING, BREAKING HEARTS

> ... we could say that most men in a concentration camp
> believed that the real opportunities of life had passed.
> Yet, in reality, there was an opportunity and a challenge. One
> could make a victory of those experiences, turning life into an
> inner triumph, or one could ignore the challenge and
> simply vegetate, as did a majority of the prisoners.
> —Viktor Frankl

KEY TOPICS

- Collective trauma
- PTSD
- Meaning-making and healing

The idea that health care professionals, and particularly nurses, might suffer from "death overload," collective trauma, and possibly PTSD has not been given much attention. For nurses who work in areas where death is a frequent occurrence, we would do well to address it. In the larger realm of things, post 9/11 and hurricane Katrina here in the United States, and globally in the wake of devastating earthquakes, tsunamis, cyclones, and ongoing horrible acts of terrorism, we know that carers must be prepared to face the possiblity of collective trauma at any time.

As I write this, the East coast is trying to recover from a deluge of flooding and losses brought here with hurricane Irene. The people of Haiti are still trying to heal from their horrific losses of 2010, and all over the world, acts of terror and natural disasters force us to collectively face death and threats of death each day. A cruise ship, the Costa Concordia, ran aground on January 13 with more than 4200 people on board and thirty-two people died. All of the people involved in every one of these events were traumatized, as were all those individuals who were involved in the rescue efforts. Indeed, as I write this I can hear my mom telling us the story of the airplane that crashed in 1960 in Park Slope. She was an RN working at Methodist Hospital in Brooklyn where the only survivor of the crash, an 11-year-old boy named Stephen Baltz, was taken, and who a day later succumbed to his injuries. I heard the story on more than one occasion while growing up—clearly indicative of the sustaining memory and horror that the event created for my mom and I am sure all of those who were working at the hospital during that time.

The following account was shared by a nurse in one of our focus group discussions:

> *This week in our nursing class on death and dying I was reminded of things that I felt were long [gone] from my memory. I was working in my EMS job on a Tuesday morning and I had just picked up my first patient in downtown Manhattan. On my way to the hospital, the Twin Towers were attacked. I remember the events of the day vaguely; what remains vivid is the sound of bodies hitting the ground all around me as people leapt from the burning buildings. I remember the smell of the mixture of burning flesh and jet fuel, and my most vivid memory is that of ashes falling all around. I was asked if I wanted to debrief, I declined . . .*

> *Eight years later I had a bad pediatric trauma. It was a little boy that was pinned between a tree and a car, causing his skull to crack open and his brain matter to spill out. Even now, as I type this, my hands are shaking. I have had hundreds of patients and deaths since then, but this seems to be the one call that still affects me. My supervisor at the time put my partner and I out of service and requested that we debrief. Critical incident stress debriefing (CISD) was readily available for us whenever we needed it, but somehow I never felt I needed it, not even then. I went home and thought I would be okay . . . . I didn't sleep for a few nights.*

> *Years later, whenever I am reminded of the friends and coworkers we lost in 9/11 or of that little boy, tears well up in my eyes, maybe I should have gone, maybe it would have helped me. I believe now that CISD is important and that it should be offered more often and by all employers, health related or not. If I had a choice today I would take advantage of the help offered. I believe that it should be explained that it is alright not to be okay after any event, whether it is a terrorist attack or a tragic and sudden death. At the end of the day when we go home, we are no longer nurses, paramedics, or doctors—we are human beings.*

This nurse became aware that she would have benefited from some treatment for the trauma she suffered. It more than likely was the number one reason why she took the class on death and dying. During classes she was able to share her feelings with others who were supportive and were able to bear witness to her anguish. I am sure it not only facilitated her healing, it helped others who might not otherwise have been willing to take advantage of CISD when it is needed and offered. Healing from traumatic experiences begins with the acknowledgement that one is hurting and it is enhanced by the efforts others make to acknowledge and support those who are suffering from the trauma.

COLLECTIVE TRAUMA

Collective trauma is when a group of people are traumatized at the same time by some thing. Whatever it is, the something is so devastating that whether or not the trauma is primary in nature does not matter to the group as a whole. *Everyone* experiences the pain and anguish together. The suffering is of a palpable nature in an entire group of people. It could be a small group, a community, or a larger group such as a society or country, or even of a global magnitude. It does not mean that the trauma is the same for everyone; some suffer more and others less. What it means, though, is that everyone is *sharing* in the horror.

For as long as humankind has been in existence, we have had events that result in collective trauma. Natural disasters and human-made disasters have been many. As a native New Yorker, I have both witnessed and experienced the devastating feelings arising from collective trauma. The events of September 11, 2001 will remain forever imprinted in the minds and hearts of people throughout the world. It was an appalling act of terrorism thrust upon innocent human beings and many people continue to suffer from PTSD related to it. For those living and working in New York City, it constituted both primary and secondary trauma. Working in the city, I can tell you it was tough stuff to enter the city in the days, weeks, and months after 9/11. To this day I cannot look at the New York skyline without welling up with tears (Todaro-Franceschi, 2011d).

In the immediate aftermath of 9/11, nearly half of the American population reported symptoms of PTSD (Schuster et al., 2001), and in the days, weeks, and months following, many continued to have symptoms of PTSD along with the fear of future terrorist attacks. I worked with one student who had lived in close proximity to the Twin Towers. She watched the events of that day unfold from her apartment window, and she continued to have symptoms of PTSD along with terrible panic attacks for a long time afterward, which affected every single aspect of her life.

Yet, I can also tell you that something occurred in New York City immediately after 9/11 that I wish we could all capture and hold in our hands and hearts and never allow to dissipate. We were *nicer* to one another. There was evidence of unity—connectedness—and purpose, the likes of which I had never seen before in my hometown and have not seen since (Todaro-Franceschi, 2011d). One can attribute it to our sense of vulnerability, but for the grace of God it could have been us or our loved ones. But in actuality, it *was* our loved ones, for we are all one. From that sense of community—the collective nature of the trauma—we were able to continue to function and for a short space of time, we were more acutely aware of our *oneness*, our *we-ness*. This sense of oneness, I believe, is what got us all through that horrible time and it is what contributed to our collective healing, not only in NYC, but throughout the United States and the rest of the world where people suffered because of the 9/11 attacks.

Depending upon the nature of the traumatic event, those who have been collectively traumatized may pull together, such as what happened in the United States and other countries that were affected from 9/11, or the event may completely fracture the social fabric of the group—community, society—because the event causes such wide-spread devastation that the group can no longer perceive themselves as a group at all, but rather a bunch of disconnected people who are all trying individually to survive.

A Loss of Communality

The Buffalo Creek disaster is a case in which it has been said that there was a loss of communality due to the nature of the collective trauma (Erikson, 1995). In 1972, a dam burst in a coal mining community, killing 125 people and physically injuring another 1,100. Over 4,000 people were left homeless. Prior to the events of that day, these people who lived in a mountainous community depended upon each other and there was an undeniable kinship. After the flooding, people who had lost everything were scattered in refugee camps, separated from the neighbors they had depended on, and instead were forced to live amid strangers. Consequently, they lost their sense of connectedness and community. An in-depth discussion of collective trauma is outside the purview of this book; however, within the context of compassion fatigue in nursing, I would like to draw attention to the following relationship.

In health care settings, whether we acknowledge it or not, collective trauma is, in a very real sense, a regular occurrence. Those who work with individuals and groups of people afflicted by disease and injury are communally traumatized all the time as they work with and bear witness to pain and suffering. In his studies of the Buffalo Creek disaster and how it affected the people, Erikson (1995) wrote about a loss of

communality that he deemed was evidenced in various behavioral manifestations. Two in particular are especially noteworthy here: demoralization and loss of connection.

Demoralization was said to have occurred as both a loss of personal
morale for those traumatized but also a loss of perceived "morale anchors"
(Erikson, 1995):

> The lack of morale is reflected in a profound apathy, a feeling
> that the world has more or less come to an end and that there
> are no longer any sound reasons for doing anything. People
> are drained of energy and conviction, not just because they
> are still stunned by the savagery of the flood but because activity
> of any kind seems to have lost much of its direction and purpose
> in the absence of a confirming community surround. They feel
> that the ground has been pulled out from under them, that the
> context in which they had worked, played, and cared for
> others has more or less disappeared. (p. 409)

It was also demoralizing for the people who suffered this collective trauma
in the sense that there had been an earlier disaster related to the same issues
and authorities had not fixed the problem, nor were these people ever
able to be fully compensated for their terrible losses. Their lives were
irrevocably changed.

The second behavioral manifestation related to the loss of communality witnessed in survivors of the Buffalo Creek collective trauma—the loss
of connection—was noted to be a sense of being separated from others to
the extent that they felt isolated and alone:

> For better or worse, the people of the hollow were deeply
> enmeshed in the tissues of their community; they drew their
> very being from them. When those tissues were stripped away
> by the disaster, people found themselves exposed and alone,
> suddenly dependent on their personal resources. . . . Many peo-
> ple feel that they have lost meaningful connection with them-
> selves. (p. 412)

I would point out that both of these behavioral manifestations (demoralization and a loss of connection), which were identified to reflect a loss of
communality as a result of collective trauma, are also prevalent in people
who are suffering from burnout. By us not acknowledging the inherently
collective traumatic nature of our work and supporting each other along
the way, we are contributing to the emotional contagion of burnout.

People who are exposed to collective trauma are at increased risk
for anxiety and panic attacks, depression, substance abuse, and the

development of PTSD. PTSD poses a particular challenge, since without treatment, it is almost impossible to heal from, but even with prompt treatment it can become chronic in nature.

POST-TRAUMATIC STRESS DISORDER

PTSD is used to describe an anxiety disorder that can emerge in anyone of any age as a response to feelings of fear, helplessness, and horror from a traumatizing event that can be either primary or second in nature. It can happen as a result of directly experienced or witnessed, life-threatening traumatic events, such as natural disasters (floods, fires, tornadoes, hurricanes, etc.), war, or terrorist attacks. It can also emerge from experiences of assault, such as domestic violence or rape. Sometimes the sudden death of a loved one can result in PTSD, too.

Veterans of war are at increased risk for PTSD, so much so that there is a Veteran's Administration National Center for PTSD. The compassion fatigue and related PTSD experienced by the carers of veterans is widespread too; the Army has its own term, "provider fatigue," for the people who develop PTSD themselves while caring for traumatized veterans (Conant, 2007). In recent years, it has become evident that family members and loved ones of veterans can also develop PTSD.

Whereas, when one is faced with danger, the normal "fight or flight" response kicks in and is a survival strategy, with those who suffer from PTSD, the response continues to exist after the danger has subsided or the traumatic experience has ended. Studied extensively, it is known to have both psychological and biological aspects—in other words—it is a transformation of the *whole*. Many people do not realize this and think the syndrome is limited to an emotional response. However, studies have shown that there are physiologic changes involved that arise from the failure of the body to respond successfully to the trauma (Yehuda, 2002a, 2002b). PTSD is often noted to be very similar to compassion fatigue, but it has a much bigger scope.

It is important to note that it is the unique aspects of each individual (physical, psychological and spiritual) that contribute to how each of us manifest signs and symptoms of suffering related to traumatic events. The diagnosis of PTSD is made when there are three distinct kinds of symptoms: reliving the event, avoiding reminders of the event, and hyperarousal (e.g., insomnia and/or impaired concentration) for a minimum of 1 month after the traumatic event (Yehuda, 2002a; see Table 10.1).

As can be seen, there is a similarity between PTSD and compassion fatigue. PTSD is most often, but not always, the direct result of someone experiencing some form of trauma, whereas compassion fatigue is usually a result of witnessing someone else's suffering. Again, what is

TABLE 10.1 Symptoms of PTSD

Revisiting the Event	Avoiding Reminders of the Event	Hyperarousal
Flashbacks, where one feels as if he or she is reliving the event	Numbness and/or detachment	Trouble concentrating
Nightmares—dreaming of the event	Disconnecting from, things seem surreal	Easily startled, more aware
Repetitive memories or thoughts	Inability to remember aspects of the event	Irritable, easily angered
Reacting to similar events	Avoiding places, people, or things that bring up memories of the event	Difficulty falling or staying asleep

traumatic for one person may not be for another; however, when the trauma is collective and effects large numbers of people, it is difficult to note whether it is primary or secondary. When New York City was attacked, one could say that every New Yorker was the victim of primary trauma, whether or not they were there that day. Some would not agree and would say that only those who were there suffered primary trauma; for those who were not there, the trauma was secondary in nature. Either way, many people all around the world developed PTSD from the events of 9/11.

Upon close examination, you might note that it is the threat to one's very existence that binds the two syndromes–compassion fatigue and PTSD—together. In cases of compassion fatigue, we co-suffer with those who are ill and/or may be facing the threat of death or are actually dying. With PTSD, be it related to individual or collective trauma, the possibility of death looms before us. Even chronic illness, in a way, threatens one's existence because it often changes one's *way* of life completely. In cases of collective trauma, the events threaten many people's ways of living–dying all at once. In all instances we hurt.

MAKING MEANING FROM TRAUMATIC EVENTS

When horrific events occur, it tests our faith in ourselves and in others. For some, it may test their religious faith as well. Very often, people who are traumatized will seek to understand how and why something has occurred. One may ask, why did it happen to him and not me? Conversely, why did it happen to me and not him? What is the meaning of this? In the larger scheme of things, is there a reason or purpose?

It is a natural human trait to seek meaning in our experiences. But as someone who claims that the universe is so ordered that there must be a purpose and reason for it all, even I have to admit, I have difficulty *finding* meaning in the many shared horrors in our history (Todaro-Franceschi, 1999, 2003). I do not understand how senseless acts of violence can occur. I do not understand why a person must sometimes suffer with incredible pain. I definitely cannot reconcile the enormous suffering I have sometimes witnessed, with any understanding of its purpose.

In 2002, three nursing faculty members at the University of Arizona, Barbara Monroe, Cheryl McGaffic, and Robin Rogers, were killed by a disturbed nursing student who then committed suicide, leaving the entire university in a state of shock and mourning. Understandably, it left the entire profession of nursing reeling, as well. I knew Cheryl and she was one of the most compassionate people I have ever encountered. It made no sense to me that nursing faculty could be killed by a student who believed himself to be so terribly alone that he felt no recourse and no remorse. But I think in instances where we cannot hope to find meaning, it is helpful to try to make meaning.

In a letter to the editor of *Nursing Science Quarterly* several years back, after the University of Arizona faculty were killed, I had written, "Yes, we can sit back and shake our heads and say what a tragedy it was. We can try to move on and act as if the whole thing was a senseless act of violence performed by a disturbed person . . . ." I went on to note that "I would like to ensure that those faculty members did not die in a senseless act of violence. I would like to make sense out of this senseless act. There are pearls of wisdom to be found and there is a lesson to be learned" (Todaro-Franceschi, 2003, pp. 184–185). Looking at repeating headlines all over the world, where people are sharing horrors and hearts are aching, I feel compelled to note that by trying to make meaning *together* we can help one another to heal.

There is a large body of literature that suggests that one's search for meaning and those activities geared toward *making* meaning out of bad experiences can help people to heal and overcome feelings of despair from traumatic experiences. The Viennese psychiatrist Viktor E. Frankl (1959) who himself survived years of horror in Nazi death camps, went on to create a revolutionary form of psychotherapy called logotherapy, which rests on the premise that our search for meaning is the driving force behind all human endeavor.

In his classic work, *Man's Search for Meaning*, he described enormous suffering and, yet, he acknowledged that even in the midst of great anguish, life has meaning and purpose in every moment that we live. Frankl (1959) noted that as human beings we have the freedom of will, and that we can will ourselves to seek and move toward making meaning in our lives. Along these lines, in a recently reported longitudinal study of what might facilitate healing for survivors from the collective trauma of the 9/11 terrorist attacks, it was found that the search for meaning helped to predict a higher stress response and incidence of PTSD, whereas *finding* meaning predicted lower PTSD symptoms (Updegraff, Silver, & Holman, 2008). I am not sure that we can always *find* meaning in everything, but I do think we can *make* meaning from anything. In instances of collective trauma it is helpful for us to support each other in the attempt to make meaning.

Collective Healing

When a group shares the horror of a traumatic event and people come together to support one another, healing is facilitated. As health care professionals we know this and encourage people who have been traumatized to seek support from their loved ones, support group networks, and so on. Yet, we often do not recognize the need for ourselves to seek the same kind of support. Having compassionate leaders who understand not only the traumatizing nature of our work, but also that we are human beings with unique characteristics is so important because every person will have different ways of dealing with the traumatizing aspects of our work based on personality, culture, and previous experiences, among other things.

In the increasing body of literature on the importance of compassion in organizations, it is repeatedly stressed that it is human beings who make up organizations—it is people who meet the goals and the mission of any work place. And we *feel*. Noted, "there is always grief somewhere in the room" when you put a bunch of people in it (Dutton, Frost, Worline, Lilius, & Kanov, 2002, p. 60). Experts in organizational behavior who have extensively studied the positive transformation that occurs when compassion is displayed by those in management note that leaders can promote compassion on two levels, by providing:

1. A context for meaning—the leader creates an environment in which people can freely express and discuss the way they feel, which in turn helps them make sense of their pain, seek or provide comfort, and

2. A context for action—the leader creates an environment in which those who experience or witness pain can find ways to alleviate their own and others' suffering (Dutton et al., 2002, p. 56).

A compassionate leader realizes that in the midst of both individual and collective trauma it is not acceptable to ask folks to come to work and put their thoughts or feelings aside. In cases of collective trauma it is especially unfitting once one realizes that healing will best take place if everyone is offered the opportunity to support and help each other.

Dutton et al. (2002) shared a story from their research on compassion in organizations; they interviewed the employees in a company where a visitor had died suddenly in the firm's hallway, even though employees had heroically tried to revive him. Afterwards the company leaders carried on business as usual, never acknowledging what had happened. They noted that it left:

> people shocked and demoralized and uncertain about how to respond should such an event occur again. Some employees were wracked with guilt over not being able to save the man's life. Others felt weak and helpless because they had no opportunity to grieve in the presence of their colleagues. They had shared a significant experience and could not console one another—or even recognize people's extraordinary efforts to revive the victim. This one event damaged not just the employees who were directly involved but also the social fabric of the whole company. (p. 57)

Notably, the managers hindered rather than facilitated employee healing, which in turn negatively affected the company as a whole.

Years ago, one of my daughters, then a high school student, volunteered to work at an AIDS Memorial quilt event in Washington, DC. I went with her, and the first moment I laid eyes on the quilt, which took up the entire space of the Mall, I was struck by the enormity of the loss—a collective loss like no other. While I had known it before—that young, old, male, and female individuals of every cultural and religious tradition have been lost to this disease, it hit me hard. Having not ever suffered a personal loss from AIDS did not matter. No one viewing that quilt was left unscathed. No one viewing that quilt could NOT be traumatized, once having seen it.

Just as compassion fatigue and burnout out are contagious, *compassion* is contagious. So why is it that we have few forums in the workplace where we can visibly share the horrors we silently witness and silently share together? I took care of that 18-month-old child with AIDs during the course of only one 12-hour shift. How many of my coworkers did that and more, and cried all night as I did? Had we the opportunity to share our compassionate caring and co-suffering, we could have consoled one another. Instead, we each carried the pain home with us and, undoubtedly, we carry the sustaining memories forever. I am sure that some of my coworkers developed compassion fatigue and still others over time burnt out.

It would seem that viewing the nature of our work with people who are suffering as a collective traumatic experience could offer us a direction for healing our wounded workforce. Research findings indicate that many people perceive benefits from traumatic experiences and that those who are able to find or make meaning following trauma are more likely to adjust and be able to live well (Poulin, Silver, Gil-Rivas, Holman, & McIntosh, 2009). Making meaning from our experiences with patients who are suffering and their loved ones can be a social benefit for all of us engaged in health care practice.

APPLYING *ART* FOR HEALING FROM SHARED HORRORS

Healing from traumatic events, be they individual or collective in nature, as with anything else, must begin with the *acknowledgement* that there is a problem. Treatment for PTSD usually entails one-to-one counseling and/ or support group therapy and frequently also requires medication for anxiety, depressive symptoms, and/or sleep disturbances. In order to *recognize* and make choices and take purposeful action to heal from PTSD, the afflicted person first has to have an understanding of the nature of the problem. For many people who are suffering with PTSD, there is so much anxiety that medication and counseling are usually the best choices that they can make initially in order to clear the way for other choices and purposeful actions. *Recognize* that PTSD is not something that we create by ourselves. It is physiologically and psychologically instigated and transforms the whole. Thus, a holistic approach is needed in identifying choices and purposeful actions for healing, and, as always the action plan will need to be finely tailored to each person. Turning outward toward self and other is of vital importance because it is difficult to heal from PTSD without therapeutic intervention. Journaling, meditation, and reconnecting with nature and with loved ones can facilitate finding meaning and instances where it may seem impossible to find meaning, we can make meaning.

ART (acknowledging, recognizing choices of purposeful actions one can take and turning outward toward self and others) can also be applied in groupwork to heal from instances of collective trauma. People who suffer from traumatic experiences can be encouraged to appreciate the meaningful connections in their moments together. We can encourage ourselves and each other in making meaning.

When people experience collective trauma, we learn that life is not always fair and that sometimes no matter how hard we try, we cannot control the events leading to changes in our lives. Dying, death, and threats of death are all integral with life and living. Yet there are always choices that we can make to move forward and to heal. Turning toward ourselves and each other, we can explore what choices we have and can make right now to help reaffirm our sense that this moment *right now* is meaningful and filled with purpose.

I have often wondered how it was that so many children imprisoned in concentration camps, drew pictures of, and wrote about, butterflies.

The very young as well as older children saw in butterflies a way to overcome some of their isolation and terror for a brief time, and they were able to describe the beauty, along with the ugliness, all the meaning and purpose of their lives, in such vivid portrayals (e.g., as have been shared in the drawings and poems from the Terezin concentration camp in 1942–1944; Volavkova, 1993). In some ways, children are smarter than adults; these children knew what no one was saying, that many of them would die. Yet, by their reflections, it is clear that many held hope for their future, while being in the moment.

Nurses can find hope for the future while being in moments where we bear witness to individual and collective trauma. We readily acknowledge when others are traumatized and are suffering. For our own quality of life, both personal and professional, it is perhaps time for us to acknowledge that we have been and continue to be collectively traumatized in our work environments. We can encourage ourselves and each other to make meaning from our collective suffering. We can turn outward toward ourselves and each other.

KEY POINTS

- Collective trauma occurs when a group of people experience a life-threatening event or bear witness to another person (or persons) experiencing a life-threatening event.
- What is traumatic for one person may not be for another.
- Working with people who have life-threatening illness or injury and are suffering can be viewed as a form of collective trauma that all health care professionals and others who work in health care settings experience together.
- PTSD is an anxiety disorder that has a biological as well as psychological basis and emerges from traumatic life-threatening experiences.
- PTSD and healing from traumatic events require one to first acknowledge that he or she has been traumatized and that an intervention of some sort is necessary.
- Healing from experiences of collective trauma is facilitated by compassionate caring and being supportive of each other.
- Healing from traumatic experiences may be facilitated by finding meaning or making meaning.

Part V

BEATING THE ODDS

*It's up to us. We can spend our lives cultivating our resentments
and cravings or we can explore the path of the warrior—nurturing
open-mindedness and courage.*
—PEMA CHODRON

Chapter 11

CULTIVATING COLLECTIVE MINDFUL AWARENESS

I think we have to transform the culture, by beginning with a
nucleus which makes a new culture. It doesn't begin with
a practice. Practice must follow out of something deeper.
—DAVID BOHM

KEY TOPICS

- Fostering collective mindful awareness
- Nursing education and leadership as instrumental for reaffirming our purpose
- *ART* for group-focused work to address issues of professional quality of life

---

To cultivate collective mindful awareness aimed at healing and preventing compassion fatigue and burnout in nursing, we need to first begin to "think in a vocabulary of oneness" (Myss, 1996, p. 286).

Researchers at the Institute of Noetic Sciences, an organization that focuses predominantly on how human beings actualize their potentials, explore what they refer to as "consciousness transformation," where one has shifts in consciousness, usually through meditative practices, somewhat akin to peak or optimal experiences (Vieten, Amorok, & Schlitz, 2006). They noted that these experiences lead one from an "I to we" way of viewing the world, a broadening of one's sense of self that has a spiritual component where one is aware of something greater than his or her self, something bigger even than "we" or "us"—it is beyond us. This, too, gets at my basic premise in the enigma of energy—we come to see that whatever we do is reflected in the whole; it is all essentially one

(Todaro-Franceschi, 1998, 1999). I am reminded of a quote from physicist David Bohm (1998) that I use often: "To see that everybody not merely *depends* on everybody, but actually everybody *is* everybody in a deeper sense" (p. 110).

Scientists can be very philosophical, and unsurprisingly (to me), very spiritual. Thus, I have never understood why many individuals in nursing believe that spirituality is not something we should refer to in our teaching, research, and practice, and that religion is better relegated to a place where it cannot infect objectivity (and science). When those such as Albert Einstein, Stephen Hawking, Paul Davies, and David Bohm, among so many others, could repeatedly and in depth reflect upon and discuss spirituality and, indeed, religion in their work, it seems almost sacrilegious for us in nursing not to do so.

There is an unquestionably inherent *spiritual* component to nursing, for spirituality is nothing more (or less) than a sense of being connected with everything and everyone else. Nurses who are *heartful*—compassion content—are those who are mindfully aware of their connectedness to others and it fuels them to be with and do for their patients.

In a discussion on science and theology, David Steindl-Rast (Capra, Steindl-Rast, & Matus, 1991) talked about how we can walk around feeling lost or orphaned and then suddenly there is a moment where everything clicks and we feel like we belong, where we think:

> "I belong to all other humans." Even if there is nobody around, this is clearly felt. I belong to all the animals, to the plants. And belonging means I am at home with them, I am responsible for them and to them. You see, I belong to them as much as they belong to me. We all belong together in this great cosmic unity. (p. 15)

In nursing, we need to cultivate and foster a collective awareness of our we-ness—our oneness—in order to enhance our professional quality of life.

A CLEAR PATH FORWARD

In nursing, we talk about and emphasize patient-centered care, patient advocacy, and of late, even patient etiquette. How do we really go about getting it to happen? The first step is for all of us engaged in the multiplicity of nursing roles to look at ourselves and at what is going on *in* nursing. Are *we* happy or content? Do we believe in ourselves individually and collectively as professionals who are important? Does our practice emulate what we emphatically note in our code of ethics, to be the values, virtues, excellences, of our profession? Are we treating ourselves and each other well? Do we support each other, mentor each other, and acknowledge each other as human beings? Are we providing the best care that we possibly can to those who need us? We need to explore these questions individually and collectively in our work environments.

Move It On Up!

From a nurse educator perspective, I see a clear path for our future workforce. In nursing education, we have an impetus to role model and teach compassion; our moral code insists that nurses both teach and learn it. Given that nurses must care for people of all races and religions, it is imperative that we have an understanding of the intricate nature of both healing and suffering from a transcultural perspective.

Nurse educators can do much to minimize and prevent the contagion of the syndromes of compassion fatigue and burnout. In schools of nursing the curricula should include compassion skills, assertiveness and advocacy training, self-care strategies, and end-of-life care—not just a dab of it here and there, at least a full course immersion of it. It should not be pot luck whether our future nurses are taught this content.

The latest literature on nursing education calls for radical transformation. In their book on the implications of the IOM reports for nursing education, nurse authors Anita Finkelman and Carol Kenner (2009) wrote in great detail about how we can use the IOM reports to guide, generate, and sustain positive change in nursing education and practice. The core competencies of providing patient-centered care, participating in interdisciplinary teamwork, employing evidence-based practice, applying quality improvement, and using informatics are quite visible (Finkelman & Kenner, 2009). Their relationship to the forces of magnetism is very clear.

In order to make it all come together, educators and leaders need to emphasize the importance of putting the oxygen mask on first. There needs to be inclusion on the development of ways to meet our needs and care for ourselves individually and collectively so that we are prepared to care for others without hurting ourselves in the process. Kenner, Finkelman, Weatherby, Long, and Kupperschmidt (2009) carefully address the many issues that our profession faces, which came out in the wash, so to speak, with Gordon's (2005) book on nursing against the odds. They note:

> We do not play well together, and this hurts us tremendously in the bigger political arena. We cannot blame all this on physicians and healthcare organizations because they can only take away as much power as we are willing to give up. (p. 255)

What has been stressed as important for nursing education in many of the recent reports does not address the needs of the *nurse*. As Kenner et al.

(2009) note, only we can do that. We have to come to terms with the fact that we can preach self-care to people, but we do not teach, practice, and live what we preach. The many intertwined issues related to the incidence of compassion fatigue, moral distress, and burnout in nursing detailed throughout this book and in the growing body of literature on these subjects mandates that we turn toward ourselves at this juncture. We simply cannot afford not to do so. The health and quality of life for *all of us*—nurses, patients, their loved ones, and, indeed, *our* loved ones—is at stake.

In 2007, when the Carnegie Foundation report on nursing education came out, spearheaded by nurse scholar Pat Benner and colleagues (Benner, Sutphen, Leonard, Day, & Shulman, 2009), a clear emphasis was placed on three apprenticeships, which all seemed to be of equal importance: (1) teaching "nurse think"—the learning of practical reasoning skills; (2) teaching skills through coaching and simulation, where clinical reasoning development goes hand in hand with skill acquisition; and (3) teaching and facilitating the development of social/moral roles and ethical behaviors. The third one seems to consistently get the short end of the stick. While nurse educators, scholars, and leaders such as Nightingale, Rogers, Carper, Liaschenko, Mason, and Benner, to name just a few, have, over the course of nursing's historical development, repeatedly advocated for our selfhood (which includes our inherent ability to compassionately care) and self-recognition, as powerful contributors in health care, the very essence of our being continues to be denied by many individuals, in, and out of, nursing.

In addition to the studies that the IOM has performed related to nursing, several other key studies have been done in recent years, which were noted in the committee report in 2009 from the Robert Wood Johnson Foundation (RWJF) Initiative on the Future of Nursing, at the Institute of Medicine. Just to mention a few, the Josiah Macy, Jr., Foundation work, *Who Will Provide Primary Care and How Will They Be Trained?* and *Continuing Education in the Health Professions: Improving Healthcare Through Lifelong Learning,* both suggest that nurses are key players in health care and that more emphasis needs to be placed on education and lifelong learning (RWJF, 2009).

The Committee on the RWJF Initiative on the Future of Nursing, at the Institute of Medicine (2009), developed a vision for a transformed health care system. To summarize the key message of their in-depth report, they noted the following:

1. Nurses should practice to the full extent of their education and training.

2. Nurses should achieve higher levels of education and training through an improved education system that promotes seamless academic progression.

3. Nurses should be full partners, with physicians and other health professionals, in redesigning health care in the United States.

4. Effective workforce planning and policy making require better data collection and an improved information infrastructure. (p. 4)

The committee emphasized that, "The education system should provide nurses with the tools needed to evaluate and improve standards of patient care and the quality and safety of care while preserving fundamental elements of nursing education, such as ethics and integrity and holistic, compassionate approaches to care" (RWJF, 2009, p. 31).

When so many intelligent groups are emphasizing our importance in achieving transformation in health care, how is it that this fundamental aspect is so frequently left out of our nursing curriculum—that in most programs we do not teach students to appreciate themselves and each other? Without having been taught that they are full partners, with physicians and other health professionals, nurses cannot expect to know that they are. The topics of ethics, integrity, and holistic compassionate approaches to care are not taught in any real depth in most schools of nursing, leaving nurses deprived of those fundamental elements that could help to sustain our individual and collective well-being while working in complex health care environments. If, and only if, we change the basic education of our future workforce, can we rise to meet the challenges in health care and the expectations of society.

In the seminal work for which Benner (1984) became so well known, *From Novice to Expert: Excellence and Power in Clinical Nursing Practice*, she expounded upon what makes a nurse an expert practitioner. Through her observations and critical analysis of nurses in practice, she offered us a clear path forward. Hard put to choose which one or two of the many thoughts and important points she offered, I think it would be helpful to our profession, if at this time, folks in nursing education and leadership who have this book were to take it down from their bookshelves, dust it off, and re-read it. Those who do not have the book should really get a copy to read; it is enlightening, to say the least. I often think that had we all taken this work to heart and mind when she wrote it, we would have transformed nursing education *radically* back then—almost 30 years ago.

In her studies, Benner (1984) identified six qualities of power inherent in the caring provided by the expert nurses she observed: transformative, integrative, advocacy, healing, participative/affirmative, and problem solving (p. 210). While space does not permit a discussion on each of them, I want to stress that all of them combined reflect the compassionate caring practices inherent in our work. Throughout her book, Benner repeatedly comes back to caring and knowing participation as foundational elements for expert nursing practice. I offer just a few of her thoughts here to reemphasize what has already been noted. Benner emphatically wrote: "... It is *not* true that the best protection against burnout lies in distancing and control strategies—that is, protection against caring" (p. 214). She shared an exemplar of a nurse who provided comfort and presence during a woman's last moments of life and noted that it:

> ... illustrates the best antidote to burnout in the work setting; engagement and involvement .... In participating, this nurse was able to use the meanings and resources inherent in this poignant event. In caring, she not only experienced pain, but also strength and affirmation. She learned first-hand about a human possibility that many never experience or witness and she felt affirmed and stronger for it. One could imagine that a detached, avoiding approach would have offered only frail protection and no positive resources such as the participative and affirmative power of caring that this nurse gained. (p. 214)

Benner (1984) also stated that the emotional component of our caring practices can lead us in meaningful ways that impersonal, disconnected caring will not. Our unique ways of knowing can make all the difference: "A preference for detached, reflective reasoning and formal explicit knowledge overlooks the role of caring with its attendant emotions—vague feelings, hunches, a sense that something is not right—or the creative search and cue sensitivity that occur as a result of caring" (p. 216). Yet, in much of the recent literature where authors stress the changes that need to take place in nursing education, there is little to indicate that any importance is being (or even should be) placed on the development of social/ moral roles, ethical behaviors, and unique ways of knowing. There is little that addresses self-care strategies for the nurse—something which is, in our code of ethics, noted to be *central* to the well-being of our profession. There is little or no mention of compassion, or caring practices, and by this I am referring to that human-to-human connection so vital to us in our practice.

Many nursing schools continue to downsize ethics content across the board in undergraduate, graduate, and doctoral programs. In some places, it has been downsized so much it is nonexistent. The social aspects that are clearly delineated in our code of ethics are visibly *invisible*. Maybe it is there and I overlooked it? But I was *looking* for it. If I cannot see it, others cannot either. The omission sticks out like a sore thumb, and that it is an ominous omission one cannot doubt.

Benner (1984) wrote that, "to abandon the power inherent in caring relationships is to sell out but, worse yet, it is to become alienated from our own identity and to thwart our own excellence .... Nursing without caring is powerful and devastating" (p. 216). If we are not selling ourselves out entirely, as Benner suggested, we are definitely selling ourselves *short*. As a result, we have a lot of unhappy nurses, increasing incivility and bullying among ourselves in our workplaces, including in academia, many people leaving nursing who should stay, and, conversely, people not coming into nursing who should. The cost to us individually and collectively as a profession is nothing compared to the cost to those we serve, those whose quality of living-dying is most assuredly in jeopardy.

So I would like to propose that we take all of this downsized and missing curricula material and move it on up to make a 6th core competency that will be listed as number 1. I am drawing a blank on what to call it, but I know at least some of what needs to be in it. The following are a good start:

- Development of a sense of the importance of nursing *as a collective body* and as the largest constituents of health care professionals involved in assuring the quality of living–dying for people.

- Development of a sense of one's own salience as a nurse engaged in providing quality caring for people during both living and dying.

- Compassion skill development that encompasses learning first how to apply it to ourselves and each other with self and group care strategies (mentoring and coaching) and then how to apply it in practice (compassion as a value, virtue, and excellence).

- Learning and applying, through knowing participation, assertiveness and advocacy skills—enough of them in order to make sure that our voices are heard!

- The identification of, and prevention strategies for, professional quality of life issues (compassion fatigue, moral distress, burnout, etc., and this includes learning how to face death and care for the dying!).

Lastly, physician Wiley Souba (2002) wrote that many of his colleagues have become "disenchanted with their ability to serve as advocates for and provide care to their patients" and that their work is ultimately less fulfilling (p. 139). He claimed that medicine needs to build dialogue on meaning and purpose into the medical curricula; I would say we need to include it in all health professional curricula. In nursing, if we take time to talk about and reflect upon the meaning and purpose of our work, we will never lose sight of the fact that it emerges from and is maintained by our connection with others.

TRANSFORMING THE WHOLE THROUGH LEADERSHIP
AND STAFF DEVELOPMENT

For our current workforce, we must look to our nurse leaders and staff development educators for guidance. The goal for leaders is always to get a group of individuals to work cohesively in attaining the overall mission of the workplace; for those of us in health care, the mission is the provision of quality health care *and* quality caring to enhance the quality of living–dying for all people. A good leader in any organization knows that in order to meet any end point, one must begin with the community of people who have to do the work, acknowledging that without those people, the work could not get done. Cultivating a communal environment is crucial, and for nurses today, perhaps more essential than ever before. Positive leadership is necessary for this cultivation, hence the need for transformational leaders.

Nurse leaders and staff development educators can identify with staff the positive and negative aspects of professional quality of life and can, through visioning and innovative thinking, facilitate and implement needed changes in the systems that are creating workforce woes. Kent (2003) wrote about finding personal meaning in a chaotic, crazy world. His message is simple; it is not what is external to us that creates our lives and gives us meaning and happiness. Instead, he noted, it depends on how we *respond* to what is outside ourselves; it is always a matter of choice and we control our inner lives. Then again, I do believe that what exists outside of us is a part of us, a part of the whole, and we never really respond to anything; we change or transform *with* everything, all together, all the time. The notion that things are separate entities is a leftover idea from Newtonian times and it just is not so. We are the *whole*—only we can make things different.

Toxic Leadership and Handlers of Toxicity

Transformational nurse leaders who identify areas where change is needed to enhance quality caring focus on the interaction between *all* of the environment and *all* of the human beings that are a part of it. Notably, to be a leader in health care today can be extremely stressful and even toxic at times. Frost, working with a colleague, Sandra Robinson (Frost, 1999a; Frost & Robinson, 1999), in his studies of organizational behavior, identified and described a phenomenon they called *toxic leadership*. They posited that there are two kinds: (1) "a form of action and practice by leaders and systems that creates pain and suffering in others and in the organizations," and, (2) "the compassionate face of leadership and its costs on the individuals who exercise it" (Frost, 1999a, p. 130).

The first type of "toxic leader" is the one who "creates pain and suffering in others and in the organizations" (Frost, 1999a, p. 130). I would call these people "managers," not leaders. They manage to make everyone miserable and they usually do it by applying *power as control* (Barrett, 2010). This manager does not capitalize on the strengths of staff; does not recognize, respect, or acknowledge their good qualities, and thus devalues their contributions to the workplace. Everyone encounters at least one of these "toxic leaders" during the course of their work life. I have certainly encountered more than a few!

The second kind of "toxic leader" is the "handler" of toxicity in the workplace. Leaders who are toxic handlers, through their compassionate caring actions, alleviate the suffering of their staff by dispersing, dissipating, or dissolving the emotional toxins in the environment (Frost, 1999a, 1999b). These are also the leaders who acknowledge and value the contributions their staff makes to the organization and they are the kind of leaders we need in nursing, the ones who lead by *power as knowing participation* and who inspire others to develop their own power as knowing participation (Barrett, 2010).

Frost pointed out that toxic handlers can, and often do, absorb the toxicity and consequently are themselves more vulnerable to emotional exhaustion. The thing is, nurse leaders are called upon to do what all *nurses* do: they need to appreciate and co-suffer with their staff as their staff, in turn, are called upon to co-suffer with and appreciate patients and their loved ones:

> When toxic handlers help others, they often ... wrap the other person's suffering in love, though they might not characterize it quite this way. To respond constructively to someone else in pain is an act of compassion, a way of reaching out to a person who is alone and suffering. Efforts to reconnect people to their competence and sense of self-worth are expressions of love. (Frost, 1999b, p. 108)

Higher-level administration has to take part in helping nurse leaders to cultivate the necessary transformational skills, which includes learning how to be an effective toxicity handler without becoming burned out themselves. One cannot understate the importance of being attentive to ourselves. The oxygen mask really does need to go on our own faces first!

Magnets, Appreciative Inquiry, and Nursing Theory

One of the underlying themes throughout the preceding pages has been an emphasis on making opportunities to appreciate ourselves individually and collectively as important contributors in health care. Appreciative inquiry is a method of research and a model for organizational change that is based on recognizing the positive strengths or aspects of others and also things in our environment (Cooperrider & Whitney, 2005). Instead of focusing on problems and trying to get to their root cause in order to fix them, with appreciative inquiry, positive change comes about from a focus on the things that we already know work. Looking at what experts in organizational change management refer to as the positive core—the assets, strengths, and resources—of a workplace, the people in a work setting come to appreciate more, and are then better able to actualize the potentials of the organization as a whole in order to meet its mission (Cooperrider & Whitney, 2005).

In health care organizations, the heart of the positive core is *us*, with our unique ways of knowing and our compassionate caring practices. That is why the Magnet model is so powerful—it acknowledges and builds on our strengths, valuing and capitalizing on the many positive aspects of nursing. I am convinced that many hospitals cannot attain Magnet status because they are still looking for the root causes of problems instead of looking at and building upon what makes things work and work well . . . WE make things work, and we get it done especially well when we are supported to do it the way we know it should be done, with both clinical competency and compassionate caring.

Appreciative inquiry is noted to make "a space in which people are free to be heard" (Cooperrider & Whitney, 2005, Kindle Location 828–33). Leaders in Magnet-designated settings tend to be strong advocates for their staff and foster an environment where nurses practice more autonomously, being given not only the responsibility and accountability for their practice, but also the authority. In these settings, nurses' voices are heard! Undoubtedly, transformational leaders in Magnet-designated hospitals are so successful because they are compassionate carers and their staff feel adequately supported.

While the idea of compassion has been around since the ancients, and there has been much discourse about it in various disciplines, up until recently there has been very little focus on the part compassion plays in organizations (Frost et al., 2006). If we reflect on this a bit in nursing, we must come to realize that in this there is an opportunity for the discipline of nursing to move forward and make great strides in health care organizations, simply because compassion is an integral part of nursing.

We have many nursing theoretic frameworks that emphasize the good—notions of caring and an ethic of care that meld together and can guide us in practice to provide quality caring and foster compassion contentment for both the carer and cared for. Many of these theories rest on the assumption that it is all one—that human beings and their environments are inextricably connected. It is no surprise that hospitals with Magnet status are also those that are able to successfully adopt a nursing theoretic framework to guide their practice. Our nurse theorists have captured the essence of nursing—as both an art and a science.

Not many students seem enthusiastic to take classes on nursing theory. However, whenever I have taught a graduate nursing theory course, I have witnessed a heightened awareness in many students regarding the meaning and purpose of our nursing work. Many share AHA! moments that occur in their practice, events they attribute to their learning of nursing theory. There is an awful lot of affirmative "nodding," especially when we get to the caring theoretic frameworks.

The Magnet movement came about while trying to address nurse retention during a time when there was a severe shortage of nurses and when new nurse attrition was high. This is once again the current state of affairs, and it is in large part due to the culture of the institutions where the important stuff—the compassion and human-to-human connection—has either disappeared or is not readily apparent and nurtured as a virtue and an excellence.

Magnet designation is achieved through the efforts of nurses and nursing, but as McClure (2011) stressed, nurses cannot do it alone. It is truly an organizational accomplishment that is attained with the full support of all the people who work in it:

> The hospital either embodies the necessary exemplary corporate culture or it does not. It is either a place in which all employees find satisfaction in their work or it is not. It is impossible for hospitals to provide a rich and rewarding environment for nurses alone. Every individual—from the CEO to the entry-level employee—affects, and is affected by, the quality of the workplace environment. (McClure, 2011, p. 6)

The Magnet model is entirely dependent upon relational factors, which, for the most part, depend for their success upon genuine human-to-human connection and compassionate caring.

As of the most recent reports, 377 hospitals have achieved Magnet status; they are obviously in the minority. In order to move toward the ideal, which we recognize Magnet status to be, we need to address the real issues related to our lack of contentment in the workplace. The cultivation of compassionate caring and the acknowledgment that it is a motivating force behind all we do in health care is utterly necessary for us to turn things around.

Recent reports from a 10-year longitudinal study that began in 2006 indicate that nurses perceive work group cohesion—"the degree to which members of a workgroup are friendly, helpful, and take an interest in each other"—to be a significant factor in the provision of quality care (Djukic, Kovner, Brewer, Fatehi, & Cline, 2011, p. 5). The researchers stressed that while we may not be able to do much about nurse–patient ratios with the increasing shortage of nurses, there is much we can do to change the work environment in order to make it more conducive to the provision of quality care. As in the past, in this study nurses noted that their relationships with physicians and procedural justice—where "people involved in implementing decisions have a say in making the decisions" (when our voices are heard!)—were also important factors in patient care (Djukic et al., 2011, p. 5).

Over and over again, research and literature point to the importance of the relational factors—that they can make or break us in our work environment. In Magnet status hospitals, where everyone has paid attention to these factors, nurses and others involved in the care of patients are content and subsequently retained, patients are satisfied, and outcomes are better. In other words . . . . quality of care is quality caring for all.

Compassion Lessons

How do we cultivate an atmosphere that will support us to do the work we do and do it in a way that gets our hearts to stay *full* instead of heavy or empty? We have to readily acknowledge and explore those things that can help us to cultivate mindful awareness in order to be able to, day after day, go to the places that scare us and still emerge joyful and content at the end of the day. There are many techniques that can help us to reconnect with and reaffirm purpose in our being in the world of nursing. I think collectively it has to begin with compassion lessons. This is not to say that we are not all compassionate people; it is rather to say that we need to reawaken that part of our personhood so that we are better positioned to emulate compassion in our day-to-day living and working. Not just expressing it to others—but also to ourselves.

Nussbaum (1996) noted that there are practical strategies that one may use to teach compassion and that this should be one of the goals of public education in order to develop the qualities of good citizenship. She stressed that those engaged in education teach and "cultivate the ability to imagine the experiences of others and to participate in their suffering" (p. 50). She went on to note the following:

> This education of the imagination should take a particular form. I have said that a crucial part of the ethical value of pity is its ability to cross boundaries of class, nationality, race, and gender, as the pitier assumes these different positions in imagination, and comes to see the obstacles to flourishing faced by human beings in these many concrete situations. (p. 51)

In nursing, while we teach cultural sensitivity, we do not aim to teach compassion in this manner. It seems to be taken for granted that nurses will place themselves in the position of their patients and try to understand their suffering. It is time to change this and make compassion lessons an integral part of the curriculum. Educators and nurse leaders can teach compassionate caring using clinical vignettes and reflective exercises.

One year I found out after the fact that several students had cheated on a pharmacology exam. According to our university policy, unless you witness and/or have documentation from others who have witnessed cheating, there is not much you can do about it. Two students came to me to tell me of the cheating; they did not give me any names and they did not want to document what they had seen. So, I thought about what I could do and came up with an imagery exercise. I walked into class the following week and asked the students to close their eyes and do the following:

> *Picture your loved one coming into the ER in a life-threatening situation. The nurse, who had cheated her way through pharmacology classes, is not all that knowledgeable about the medications that should be administered in this instance, and as a result, she gives the wrong medication or the wrong dose. Consequently, your loved one codes and winds up in a vegetative state.*

I left the rest to their imagination. Noticeably, quite a few students were in tears, and I like to think that imagery exercise created a sustaining memory for many students, which occasionally resurfaces to remind them to always consider that the actions they take will have consequences for others.

Nurse theorist Myra Levine (1972) shared a poignant story of how her life and nursing career evolved over time. Trained when nursing was still definitely considered gendered labor, she noted the basic technical skills that nurses had to develop and how she excelled at learning and practicing them. She shared how she gave birth to her first child, and when waiting for her newborn son to be brought to her, she realized something must be wrong. She asked and then begged for her son. The nursery supervisor who "had no time" finally came by to tell her there was just a little mucous and he would be brought in later (p. 137). The next time she saw her son, he was dead. She described how the grief (both hers and the staff's) was so palpable:

> I could not see their sorrow from within my own, and they could not reach through to mine. They could not come, in silence, to stand beside me and share my grief. They could not watch the tears, and so I could not weep in my bewildered need not to offend them. They came to me smiling and left hurt and frightened from the mirror of my sorrow. Beyond that door was still the joy they daily lived amidst, and soon they came through it to me only when they had to come. (p. 137)

Levine (1972) went on to share how the death of her newborn son contributed to a change in her nursing practice and her development of
compassion:

> Out of my own torn spirit I had learned that I could not offer
> only a part of what I was to nursing. The cautious selection
> that allowed me to share only a small part of myself with the
> patient left us both deprived. Unless my humanity could
> speak to him, his could never flourish. (p. 137)

With her terrible loss, Levine learned that nursing has to be more than
a technical skill set. We need not (and should not!) learn this lesson through
horrific personal experiences. We can learn or, in cases where burnout has
occurred, relearn how to feel and express compassion, and we can teach it
by sharing our stories and by taking time to reflect upon them. It is time to
do so. Our individual and collective contentment depends on it. Society
depends on it.

APPLYING *ART* TO CULTIVATE COLLECTIVE AWARENESS

To reiterate, each step of *ART* can be looked at separately or together. It is all
intertwined and all steps need to be ongoing. At this juncture, I hope ART
has helped to frame a *wholistic* (not *hole*, the *whole*!) picture of what we need
to do to heal. We need to acknowledge individual and collective feelings—
make known the unknown about ourselves and one another. We need to
acknowledge what makes us happy and ensures a sense of meaning and
purpose in our work, and then we need to recognize what choices we
have that can move us in the direction we need to go. Once we have outlined all the choices, we can develop a purposeful action plan. We can
turn toward ourselves and each other and make whatever we want to
happen, happen!

Step 1: Acknowledge Feelings

In order to heal from compassion fatigue and enhance professional quality
of life, we need to work on it individually and collectively; it will not
happen alone. Anyone can make copies of Stamm's ProQOL (2010) tool
and pass them around at work (see Appendix A). Educators and leaders
can make the time for everyone to reflect on collective wounds in the workplace, knowing that a lack of acknowledgement can transform into poor
productivity, job dissatisfaction, and burnout.

With the knowledge that how we feel *cannot* be removed from our
workplace, and that our individual and collective feelings count in our

efforts to provide care, we must accept the reality that pain and anguish exists everywhere, including in the workplace. If one views civility the way nurse Cynthia Clark (2010) defined it, as "an authentic respect for others that requires time, presence, willingness to engage in genuine discourse and intention to seek common ground," then perhaps a lack of acknowledgement of another's suffering is actually incivility in disguise. Clark went on to note that, "Civility matters because treating one another with respect is requisite to communicating effectively, building community and creating high-functioning teams. Without civility, we miss opportunities to really listen and understand other points of view." Unless we make an effort to know the unknown about others in our environment, we cannot begin to understand why they may act the way they do. Some people might have good cause to be miserable, but no one has good cause to be cruel and uncaring.

Have a *Wit* day, a *Patch Adams* day, or a *Tuesdays with Morrie* day. Check out "YouTube" for clips from these and other motion pictures that poignantly capture what it means to feel compassion (and what it can do when one tries to flick the shutoff switch). Show one or two short clips at a staff meeting or in class and have a focused group discussion on key points (or, alternatively, ask participants to jot down their feelings about the clip and reflect upon them later).

Practice saying "ouch" collectively. Recall the motion picture film *E.T.: The Extra-Terrestrial*, where the boy and E.T. are so inextricably connected that whatever one feels, the other feels. Each of them displays compassion for the other—they cannot help but do so. Through their compassionate caring, each is able to facilitate the healing of the other. Being able to say ouch collectively means that you have to see things you might not normally see (or that you haven't been acknowledging)—becoming more mindfully aware. It also means that you have to go to places you normally avoid, and perhaps even the places that scare you.

Appreciating our moments exercise

Share, or if you are a nurse leader or educator, have your frontline nurses share, stories of their *caring moments* (Watson, 1999). Offering opportunities to share these moments not only shows recognition of their value, it also serves as teaching moments for other staff who may be distancing themselves for whatever reason. Whenever and wherever you can, build opportunities for storytelling of caring moments into the work environment.

Step 2: Recognize Choices and Take Purposeful Action

Some of the things that can be done to foster a community of caring include having sessions for focused group discussion on feelings concerning the workplace environment. Build in time to make known the unknown

about each other. This would include discussions regarding areas of difficulty as well as areas that are conducive to one's well-being. Bitching sessions can be very beneficial; however, they can also be time-wasting. Far
better to focus on the positive aspects of the environment and try to build
upon them, than it is to spend too much time discussing the negative.

"Hear you, hear me" listening exercise

I learned the following listening exercise many years ago at a workshop on
effective communication, and I use it in classes to teach active listening.
When I was in nursing management I also used it with staff. Those who
may think that they are great listeners are often quite surprised to find
that they are not as good at it as they thought. Listening is a skill that can
be taught and learned.

- Choose a partner. For 5 minutes one person should talk—sharing
  some important experience in his or her life. To also work on the
  development of compassion skills, you can ask the person to
  share a loss of some kind—it does not have to be the death of a
  loved one; it can be any loss. During the 5 minutes one person is
  speaking, the other person must do nothing but listen. Those who
  are listening are not allowed to speak at all. At the end of the
  5 minutes, have them switch places; the person being listened to
  becomes the listener and the other person gets to share a meaningful experience or loss. After the second 5 minutes is up, go around
  the room and have everyone share how they felt when they were
  listened to, and alternatively, how they felt when they listened. If
  there is not enough time to go around the room, have everyone
  reflect upon and later write down the following:

  > I felt . . . when I was listened to.

  > I felt . . . when I listened.

- Post their responses anonymously in the nursing lounge or on the
  course board. Have a discussion about them at your next meeting
  (or class).

Caution: Some folks have a *really* hard time with this exercise.

"I see me and I see you" exercise

This exercise, which I have arbitrarily named here, is an adaption from
Melodie Chenevert's (1988) shared gold mine of assertiveness training techniques. In a staff meeting (or a class), have everyone jot down one personal

thing about themselves (e.g., I like to garden, and I love butterflies!), one good thing they like about themselves, and then one good thing they like about the person sitting on their left. Afterward, have each person in turn, going around the room, share how they felt when asked to do this and what they wrote about themselves and their colleague.

I have found that this exercise is a real eye opener. First off, a lot of us have difficulty choosing one personal thing to share about ourselves and we have even more difficulty identifying and articulating things that we think are *good* about ourselves. More often than not, nurses will identify relational things such as "I'm kind," "I care about people," "I'm respectful of others," "I'm sensitive," and so forth. Many of us define ourselves by the way we connect with, and care for, others. It is a nurse thing and it goes back to that "nurse culture" I alluded to early on.[1] Much less often you will get someone who says, "I am intelligent," "creative," "resourceful," "objective," etc. While doing this exercise, some participants will also be surprised to find that they do not know all that much about one another (Chenevert, 1988, noted this too). So, having your staff or students do this exercise has the added benefit of helping everyone get to know and appreciate one another.

We need to do appreciative inquiries into our "we-ness." Collective work can be done to get to know the unknown about each other and find common ground. The dictate that we cannot bring our home to work and vice versa is baloney. We are human beings and our luggage goes with us. We need to embrace it—carry it along, but at the same time, acknowledge that it need not get so into the moment that it unwinds that moment enough to make it meaningless.

Do a CQI activity on compassion contentment!

When I was in nursing administration, total quality management (TQM) and continuous quality improvement (CQI) first came into being. With TQM, the organizational systems are explored from a multidisciplinary perspective and issues are supposed to be addressed as a whole, *by the whole.* Blame is not placed (or not supposed to be placed) on any one discipline or system because it is acknowledged that everything feeds into everything else.

The basic premise of TQM fits with my basic philosophy—it is all one. I led many successful CQI team efforts in my time. Perhaps what is needed in our health care world today is a systemwide (very big!) CQI, which focuses primarily on compassion for the cared for *and* the carers, a CQI that explores the issues that feed into productivity, recruitment, and retention of the carers, as well as quality and safety of care for the patients—you know, the *whole*, everything together. Things that might be explored would evolve around compassion contentment for everyone, and in this

way we could spruce up the quality of care rendered *and* quality of professional life at the same time. Nurse leaders are well positioned for this
kind of work, since they are always concerned with workforce productivity
and quality of care.

Maslach and Leiter (1999) identified six key areas for employee happiness: (1) a manageable workload, (2) a sense of control, (3) the opportunity
for rewards, (4) a feeling of community, (5) faith in the fairness of the workplace, and (6) shared values (p. 50). Taking each in turn, both staff and
leaders can reflect upon the work environment and come up with a purposeful action plan to improve any areas that are less than optimal. All are
self-explanatory, but I would draw attention to the feeling of community—once again a clear reference to our connectedness.

Encourage yourself and others to burn brightly

I am always looking for ways to enourage a passion for nursing in students,
and when I was in nursing management I looked for ways to empower and
encourage staff. I have been known to play songs during classes and staff
meetings—like the song sung by Yolanda Adams in *Honey* titled, "I
Believe . . .," or for laughs, the classic "I Can't Get No Satisfaction," or my
favorite inspirational song entitled, "What A Wonderful World," sung by
"Satchmo"—Louie Armstrong. Role-playing also works. Today there are
a slew of games and resources available in cyberspace. Be creative;
engage yourself and one another (Check out the resource section for
more information)!

You can brainstorm with coworkers to come up with creative strategies that address the need for both patients and carers to connect. Years
ago, for instance, at many places there was an overlap of shift time, like
the 3:30 to 11:30 shift had to report at 3:15 for a 15-minute overlap
during which time report was given. How about an hour overlap for
some of the staff, where the hour would be for the nurse coming on to
spend that time sitting with each patient (and or family) while the other
nurses wrapped up the shift and then gave report after the first nurse
had spent time with the patients?

Step 3: Turn Outward Toward Self and Others

After 9/11, I began an initiative to create a butterfly memorial garden on
our campus. People ask me all the time, why butterflies? They ask why I
talk so much about them and why my office is full of butterfly parapherna-
lia. People who come to my home in the spring and summer months might
find a caterpillar (or several) climbing up my walls, having escaped their
temporary safety pen, and they will surely see many different kinds of butterflies in my gardens.

Butterflies, as I have already mentioned, are a perfect representation of purposeful energy transformation, a sign of renewal, and through their continual metamorphosis, a symbol of everlasting change. Many people of different cultural backgrounds believe that the butterfly is their dead loved one come back to life in another fashion. It is a beautiful creature of nature and, to me, the most magnificent.

In a novel, *The Butterfly's Daughter*, written by Mary Alice Monroe (2011), the protagonist shares a memory of her grandmother—her *Abuela*—taking her to the park. Abuela would say to her, *"Look there! Watch them. See how people smile when they see a butterfly? They can't help themselves. Butterflies are joy with wings"* (Monroe, 2011, p. 154). I too have observed that when people notice a butterfly they smile. Yet, it has never ceased to amaze me how many people do *not see* butterflies. They are not aware of the fact that they fly about us all the time, occasionally even getting trapped in a car or a home.

Obviously I cannot seem to separate my passion for butterflies from my work life, and getting the students involved in the butterfly memorial garden has been a delight for me. I have been known to do an impromptu lesson on raising butterflies now and then in class and will even pass around a milkweed leaf with a caterpillar on it! So, it is unsurprising that my enthusiasm is a bit infectious; for example, one of my students emailed me from the school library during final exam cram time. He said, "Before I had you for a teacher, I never noticed butterflies. Now I see them everywhere. There is a butterfly right now fluttering about in the library; it made me smile."

Do you notice the butterflies? I once went to Costa Rica on vacation and one of my main goals was to see a blue morpho butterfly in the wild. I had only seen them in man-made conservatories before and I cannot tell you how marvelous it was to see them flying about in their natural habitat. It struck me that there were many natural happenings going on that other tourists and even native Costa Ricans did not seem to notice. Like the white-faced monkeys flitting from tree to tree and the egret I saw communing with a horse in a field, or the poisonous but oh so colorful dart frogs blending in with their surroundings; I could go on and on, but you get the point. We can make the opportunities to see things we normally do not see and, in so doing, reconnect with ourselves and others. We can reaffirm our sense of belonging to the universe and each other.

Individually and collectively we can seek to make meaning. We know what the purpose of our work is; we can be passionate about it together. Maisel (2005) notes that passionately making meaning is a skill that can be learned. He lists a number of things we can do in order to develop it:

> First, you need to decide how you will lead your life .... You decide to matter, to live a principled, creative, active life in

support of your cherished ideals, to manifest your potential, to do
good work, in short, to make your life meaningful .... (p. 20)

He goes on to emphasize that we can *intend* to make meaning when we
establish what our life purposes are and keep them ever present in our
awareness as we go about living. In nursing, we need to hold and maintain
the intention to fulfill our purpose as compassionate carers.

KEY POINTS

- We need to cultivate and foster a collective awareness of our
  we-ness—our oneness—in order to enhance our professional
  quality of life.
- The oxygen mask has to go on our face first; nurses need to learn
  how to show compassion to self as well as others, assertiveness
  and advocacy training, self-care strategies, and end-of-life care.
  The inclusion of these things in education will help us develop
  ways to meet our needs and care for ourselves individually and collectively, so that we are prepared to care for others without hurting
  ourselves in the process. The health and quality of life for *all of us*—
  nurses, patients, their loved ones, and, indeed, *our* loved ones—is
  at stake.
- Making time to see things we do not normally see is healing.
  Leaving our own pain and suffering behind when we go to work
  (or when we leave work) is an unrealistic expectation. We need
  to acknowledge and support ourselves and each other as human
  beings. We can make known the unknown about each other,
  which will foster a more healthy work environment.
- We need to *believe* that we are full partners, with physicians and
  other health professionals in the health care system.
- There needs to be time for us to talk about and reflect upon the
  meaning and purpose of our work, so that we do not lose sight of
  the fact that it emerges from and is maintained by our connection
  with others.

ENDNOTE

1. Some might say it is more a female thing. See Carol Gilligan's (1982)
   classic work, *In A Different Voice*, where she reflects on the way
   women think and act in relational terms.

Chapter 12

IMAGINE IT AND ACTUALIZE IT

> *"You see that old shack down there?" Lou looked at a mud-chinked,*
> *falling-down log cabin . . . . "Louisa told me about a story your father*
> *wrote when he was a little boy. It was about a family that survived*
> *one winter up here in that little house. Without wood, or food."*
> *"How'd they do it?"*
> *"They believed in things."*
> *"Like what? Wishing wells?" she said with scorn.*
> *"No, they believed in each other. And created something of a*
> *miracle. Some say truth is stranger than fiction. I think that*
> *means that whatever a person can imagine really does exist,*
> *somewhere. Isn't that a wonderful possibility?"*
> —(BALDUCCI, 2000, P. 233).

KEY TOPICS

- Imagination as a vehicle for change
- Our importance, our power
- A reiteration of how we can reaffirm our purpose

In the preceding chapters I have highlighted the many things in our chaotic and apparently broken health care system that contribute to diminished professional quality of life, and in particular, compassion fatigue and the related syndrome of burnout in nursing. Can the broken health care system be fixed? I answer in the affirmative; our health care system was created by humans and it has fallen apart because of us, so we can certainly fix it. But we can only do so by acting in concert, together. Nurses, as the largest constituents in the health care system, can lead the effort to fix things, and in places where Magnet status has been attained, nurses are the ones who have led the efforts to make the ideal become the reality. However, in order to proceed we need to get that oxygen mask on ourselves first.

Our profession as a whole needs healing and it is *ours* to heal. The many, many nurses who are compassion fatigued, morally distressed, and/or burned out, along with the bullied (and the bullies), need to turn toward themselves and one another. It is up to us nurses to turn things around in order to move forward as primary transformers. Remen's (1996) words on the nature of healing are so applicable here:

> The healing of our present woundedness may lie in recognizing and reclaiming the capacity we all have to heal each other, the enormous power in the simplest of human relationships; the strength of a touch, the blessing of forgiveness, the grace of someone else taking you just as you are and finding in you an unexpected goodness. (p. 217)

As I sit here wrapping up this book, I have just read the most recent Medscape news headlines: "One Fourth of ICU Clinicians Report Inappropriate Care" (Hand, 2011). The article highlights the findings of a survey of ICU nurses and physicians done in Europe and Israel. Of course, it points out that many of these clinicians suffer from moral distress; but just how many of them are compassion fatigued and over time will burn out, one can only imagine. And once again, as seems so often these days, the top three most read articles (by nurses) on Medscape have to do with bullying, incivility in the workplace, and nursing education.

Perhaps, as Gordon (2005) noted, nurses are working against the odds, yet as I point out, to some extent it appears that *we* are the ones creating the odds (that we are working against). We need to remember we are all essentially one. We are irrevocably connected in a manner that is often camouflaged in our places of employment, but if we remain cognizant of our inseparable nature, we can still provide caring presence despite a seemingly negative work environment, and in so doing change it for the better (Todaro-Franceschi, 1999). I believe that we are here on purpose; we each chose nursing, a health care profession, to make a difference in the lives of others, and that we do this on a day-to-day basis whether we acknowledge it or not, and that we can always strive to do it better, *on purpose.*

IMAGINE "WHAT IF"

In their book, *Imagination First*, authors Eric Liu and Scott Noppe-Brandon (2009) share some ostensibly simple but really quite profound insights regarding the importance of imagining and constructing new realities. They make a case for imagination to come first in any attempt to create change and emphasize how our imagination can fuel creativity and innovation. They define *imagination* as the:

> capacity to conceive of *what is not*—something that, as far as we know, does not exist; or something that may exist but we simply cannot perceive. It is the ability to conjure new realities and possibilities: in John Dewey's words, "to look at things as if they could be otherwise." (p. 19)

Asking "what if" requires courage. Liu and Noppe-Brandon note that it is scary because, "What if encompasses not only the possibility that the world is round and circumnavigable but also the possibility that it is flat and drops off abruptly to Hell" (p. 33).

Taking all of the preceding into consideration, it seems clear that imagination is required to move us forward. We have to imagine a different way from what currently is. We have to, as Dewey noted, *look at things as if they could be otherwise*. With our collective knowledge and our nursing talents and skills, we *can* make things be otherwise. Take, for example, the case of Joe, the patient who might have slept the rest of his life away with a medication patch on, were it not for us questioning "doctors orders." We can take what is, and what has been, and make it better. With our intelligence and nursing knowledge—our unique ways of knowing—of how it should be, we are extremely well equipped.

We all have the ability to imagine a different way—and the ability to hold a picture in our minds to guide us as we actualize our potential, collectively. Liu and Noppe-Brandon (2009) help us by outlining the following list of capabilities:

- Noticing deeply – identifying and articulating layers of detail through continuous interaction with an object of study

- Embodying – experiencing a work through your senses and emotions, and physically representing that experience

- Questioning – asking "Why" and "What if?" throughout your explorations

- Identifying patterns – finding relationships among the details you notice, and grouping them into patterns

- Making connections – linking the patterns you notice to prior knowledge and experience (both your own and others')

- Exhibiting empathy – understanding and respecting the experiences of others

- Creating meaning – creating interpretations of what you encounter, and synthesizing them with the perspectives of others

- Taking action – acting on the synthesis through a project or an action that expresses your learning
- Reflecting and assessing – looking back on your learning to identify what challenges remain and to begin learning anew. (p. 38)

WE CAN MAKE IT HAPPEN

What can be imagined *can* become reality. What do you imagine? As an educator, I imagine the day when an elective course offering such as *Changing the Face of Death* will become required for all undergraduate nursing students, when compassion lessons are a main part of the curriculum, and during clinical practicums students will be expected to also practice developing their compassion skills in addition to medication administration, wound care skills, and the like.

I imagine the day when there need be little fear that *my* nurse (or your nurse) will show compassion along with clinical skill competency, because not only does she (or he) have the time for it, having had compassion time built into the acuity level for staffing along with the technical aspects of care, but also because she (or he) *absolutely insists* on doing it—knowing it will be good for her or him as well as the people she (or he) is caring for.

I imagine the day when nurses, and especially advanced practice nurses—NPs and CNSs, will *always* feel and be able to say "nope, we are not doing it that way—we are doing it our way, because we know our way works better (and that day is coming fast!). It will only take consensus among *us*, for as I have noted, it is nursing that makes the health care system work (or not work) at all!

What do you imagine? Imagining a rebuilt New Orleans in Antieau's (2008) story, the protagonist Ruby notes:

> People rebuild the houses here to use the sun to power them. There's a whole lot of jobs created just to make these houses . . . . I can see it. Can you? . . . And there's no more poor people. Not because they goes to live somewheres else. No! Everyone has jobs they likes and cares about. They have work that inspires and heals them. They have homes of beauty . . . . I can see it. I can see the parties and the food and the laughter and the love. I loves, loves, loves it. Can you see it? Can you feel it? Can you make it happen? Yes, yes, yes. This will be the Place Where We Renewed the World. I tapped my chest. "Right here." I looked around. "Right in all of us." (p. 195)

Imagine. Right now this can be the place where we—nurses—heal ourselves and reaffirm our purpose, and in so doing, renew the health care world. . . . Right here, right in all of us.

Having explored the many facets of compassion fatigue and burnout, it is hoped that readers now recognize their own vulnerability as well as that of their staff and coworkers. Lee Shulman (2009), president emeritus of the Carnegie Foundation for the Advancement of Teaching (Benner, Sutphen, Leonard, Day, & Shulman, 2009), reflected:

> ... when I think about the preparation of nurses, I see key elements of preparing lawyers and teachers, engineers and ministers, physicians and psychotherapists, social workers and institutional managers. The work is physically grueling and intellectually taxing. It is both routine and filled with the unexpected and the surprising. Nursing education is preparation for remarkably hard work .... Nursing is indeed a hybrid profession, an interdisciplinary and interprofessional nexus of roles and obligations. At its core, however, remain the expectations for caring and for advocacy, for ministering to the needs of those who are ill. Hybrids are often particularly robust because they combine the strengths of several species into one. But they may also be particularly vulnerable.
>
> *—Kindle location, 148*

We cannot eradicate or overcome our vulnerability; however, by recognizing that we are all one, nurses can work together to transform the quality of living-dying for everyone.

Individually and collectively, we can heal from and/or avert compassion fatigue and the related syndrome of burnout. Nurses are natural warriors. Not warriors in the ways of aggression, but rather warriors of nonaggression—people who bear witness to the suffering of others and try to alleviate it. Chodron (2001) noted that these warriors—the bodhisattvas—are people who "hear the cries of the world" and are willing to train "in the middle of the fire," meeting challenges that take unbelievable courage and perseverance to overcome, and doing so despite sometimes enormous degrees of discomfort to oneself (p. 5).

Caring for a 4 year old with multiple trauma who is clearly dying, and bearing witness to not only that child's suffering but also that of his family members, takes colossal courage. Sitting with a woman during the night who is in terrible pain with advanced cancer, knowing she will not live to see her children reach adulthood, sharing her life story, her hopes and regrets, or, holding an 18-month-old who is dying of AIDS, never having really lived; these are no simple tasks. Standing up to a physician (or anyone for that matter) who does not respect what you bring to the health care world—saying no, this is not right, or we can do it better—these are all acts of the warrior, the bodhisattva.

EVERYONE IS A VIP AND HAS THE RIGHT TO BE!

Recently, I had the misfortune to need surgery once more, this time for gall-bladder disease. I again chose the surgeon carefully. Pre-admitting snags the day of surgery almost convinced me to turn around and go home. The nurse who took my vital signs and admitting history was curt, and at times downright rude; it seemed apparent that she hated her job. The nurse who came to start my IV told me her entire family medical history as she fished around for quite a while in the same puncture site for a vein, until I finally requested she remove the needle and start from scratch.

Post-operatively I was extremely nauseated (this time it was nausea!) and the two nurses I had to depend on during my brief 4-hour sojourn in ambulatory recovery were travel nurses. I made a point of telling them at the onset that I was a nurse, since I had not done this the last time I was in a hospital and I was rather hoping it might make this experience a bit more positive. Though both were efficient, I very clearly overheard one tell the other that she, "couldn't stand caring for patients who told her they were nurses or physicians," because, she said, "they want to be treated as VIP's." I thought at the time that she was really saying this for my benefit since she made no attempt not to be overheard. The thing is, I have never believed that any one person is more important or more entitled to quality health care (or anything else for that matter) than another. It was my feelings of both fear and vulnerability related to memories of my previous hospitalization experience that had motivated me to speak up about being a nurse.

As an educator, I am always looking for teachable moments that arise in our experiences. I have used this story in classes to get at the fact that we are all vulnerable, even if we are health care professionals. One day the majority of us will take at least one turn in a hospital bed. Having thought about her comment no small amount, I have the following rejoinder as both a patient *and* as a nurse. I do not want to be treated as a "very important person," a VIP. I want to be treated as I would treat you. I want to be treated as if I were one of your loved ones, for that is how I would most assuredly treat you, and that has always, always, been my mantra during my 30-year nursing career.

I do not want to make any excuses for my fellow nurses. Having a tough shift, week, or month just is not a good enough excuse for any of us to provide *dis*passionate and, on occasion, substandard care. In nursing, to *care* must mean to look at the whole, not the parts. Human beings are living things, not inanimate objects; a patient is not an IV, a Foley, a dressing change, or a set of vital signs. I want to reiterate that we have an autonomous practice and that we are never *ordered* to do anything. We provide care, when it is prescribed, because *we* believe it is the *right* care to assist in healing. There is power in numbers and we are many. In concert we *can* ensure that the care provided to people is not only the most knowledgeable but also the most compassionate care we can muster.

In the motion picture *Patch Adams* there is a line that goes something like this: "I want the knowledgeable prick … not the clown." Well, I for one would rather the compassionate clown who is knowledgeable, instead of a dispassionate, albeit knowledgeable professional. I want the person who treats me as a person, not an inert object. I want the person who will advocate for me and who wants to participate in my healing. I want all of this for all people; *we are all VIPs*. To that end I will continue to remind colleagues, nurses, and physicians, alike, to think carefully before acting and to continually ask your selves, "Would I be providing this care, in quite this same manner, if this person were my loved one?" I invite my colleagues to try this line whenever you witness someone providing care dispassionately. Together we might all renew our purpose in health care.

Speaking Up

One of the repeating themes throughout this book that I would draw attention to here has been the notion of *speaking up*. About a decade ago the Joint Commission (2011) began a great initiative called "Speak Up." These days there are signs on the walls in many facilities encouraging recipients of health care to *speak up* if they do not see their health care providers washing their hands, or if they have concerns about treatments. Folks are being told to pay attention to the care that they are being provided. Patients are given key points to help prevent the occurrence of errors in health care as follows:

- Speak up if you have questions or concerns.
- Pay attention to the care you get—make sure the treatments you receive are the right ones.
- Educate yourself about your illness.
- Ask a trusted family member or friend to be your advocate.
- Know what medications you take and why you take them.
- Use health care facilities that have been checked out.
- Participate in all decisions about your treatment (Joint Commission, 2011)

If your hospital has adopted a "Speak Up" or another such initiative to help safeguard patients, you need to reflect upon whether or not your facility is really living it or just paying lip service to it. It is ironic that we can have overt signs and guidelines encouraging people to speak up while health care providers (not just nurses) often seem to become quite annoyed with patients and/or families who do speak up. Indeed, far too frequently, when colleagues—nurses and physicians—or their loved ones are the recipients of care and they speak up, even they are treated by their health care providers—colleagues—as if they are a threat or a nuisance or both. Is not their advocacy for themselves or their loved ones in our best interests too? Do we not all want the same thing? We are saying we want our patients to speak up, and then when they do so, we take offence.

From the many years of listening to horrible stories from other patients and families, including nurses and physicians, I can tell you that it seems like many places do not want anyone to speak up. People are oftentimes made to feel as if they are burdens; it seems to be a commonly voiced complaint of patients and their loved ones, who, as a result, many times feel that they cannot voice any concerns to their health care providers. Yes, family members, and especially those who might seem to "know too much," can appear to get in the way sometimes. Yet, more often than not, what they have to contribute to the care we are rendering can help us to meet the goals of care, if only we would take the time to pay attention and listen to them. In order to fix our health care system we need to develop the idea of *speaking up* a little bit better. In today's lingo, we cannot just talk the talk, we need to walk the talk.

Not only should patients and their loved ones speak up; as I have said throughout the preceding pages, nurses must speak up too. The system does not and will not work well without us; *we* are the superglue that holds it all together, and if we stand firm, we can actualize whatever potentials we can envision. We need not give up our values, our compassion, our goals of care, our ethic. We can say no, this is not right, and this does not work. If we mobilize together as one, while we still may not be able to have a utopia in health care, we will be able to work collectively in a state of contentment, at least most of the time. We can work *heartfully* together.

Reaffirming purpose in nursing and healing our wounded workforce will undoubtedly and positively transform health care, for, "Healing in its essence is about breaking through the fears associated with life—fears that we don't want to face—and finding our own special inspiration, a vision of the future, that we know we're here to help create" (Redfield, 1996, p. 66). If we can regain our passion and become re-enchanted, it will be a win-win for all.

In nursing we have such a vast opportunity; how many people get to participate in the unceasing dance of human life and death on such a large scale? To bear witness to another's suffering, to be with people during both birthing and dying experiences, and everything in between, all of it is such an honor. We have a moral responsibility to do it right. We have a moral responsibility to do it right, not just for those we care for, but for ourselves as well!

Make This Time Our Tipping Point

As I come to the closing, I find myself thinking about tipping points and choices. Gladwell (2000) wrote that:

> There is more than one way to tip an epidemic .... Epidemics are a function of the people who transmit infectious agents, the infectious agent itself, and the environment in which the infectious agent is operating. And when an epidemic tips, when it is jolted out of equilibrium, it tips because something has happened, some change has occurred in one (or two or three) of those areas. (pp. 18–19)

It is up to us, individually and collectively, to turn this epidemic around. It is our choice.

We can choose to overlook rather than acknowledge there is a problem and we can continue to allow it to get increasingly out of control. Or we can accept that there is a problem and do something about it. We can allow our admirable profession to have a reputation for bullying and incivility, and we can discourage all the "would be" wonderful nurses right out of it. Or we can get to the crux of the matter and stop this behavior, getting help for the bullied *and* the bullies. We can support and encourage our young so that the "would-be nurses" know that they will be supported to become the wonderful nurses we know they can be. I think we all would rather that our profession does not have a reputation for bullying and incivility. It is far better for us to remain pictured beside those physicians and kittens as the epitome of compassion. Far better, too, for us to remain at the top of the Gallup pole, where we have been for many years and where we rightfully belong.

In a formula for leading change with RBC models, Koloroutris (2004) notes that we need to understand five key conditions—"the 5 C's"—that support our ability to participate in change: clarity, competency, confidence, collaboration, and commitment (pp. 9–10). While compassionate caring is notably evident in RBC models of care and thus one may think it is subsumed into any depiction of competency in the profession of nursing, for the purpose of understanding and emphasizing its importance, we could make it a standalone 6th "C."

Each of us has butterfly power. As we work, we *can* ditch the robot-like action and reconnect with ourselves and others. We can mind our moments and make them meaningful. For as the saying goes, we will not pass this way again—the moments with patients and their loved ones, just as those we spend with colleagues and loved ones, count and can be joyful, *heartful* moments. We *can* speak the mantra, "I will not die an unlived life." *Live* the mantra as Dawna Markova (2000), renowned inspirational writer and speaker, encourages in her poem and book of wisdom. She beseeches us to live on purpose, to explore ways to make contributions to our world that fulfill and renew us.

According to one of our most fearless warriors in nursing, Diana Mason (1999), whose voice is often heard, "power can be shared without sacrificing progress" (p. 8). She noted that there are two ways to lose power: "let others take it from us" or "become fragmented and self-destruct" (p. 8). There is power in numbers. It is really all about having "power with" rather than "power over." It is about actualizing our potential assertively and collectively through knowing participation rather than aggressively, in acts of power as control (Barrett, 2010). We need to teach it, preach it, and live it. The time to do so is now.

Eugene Peterson (1994), a Presbyterian pastor, professor, and author, shared some insightful thoughts concerning why there is a crisis in care: "Instead of being cared for people find themselves abused, exploited, organized, bullied, condescended to, and ripped off" (pp. 66–67). It is noted that the crisis of care we find ourselves in seems to have developed from:

> Something . . . subtle and pervasive, and far more likely to involve the well-intentioned rather than the ill-willed. In order to do something about it, it is not enough to get rid of a few bad eggs in our respective professions. Something like a renovation of the imagination is required—a re-visioning of who we are and what we are doing that recovers the essential sacredness of all vocational caring . . . . (p. 67)

We have to first begin by re-visioning and appreciating ourselves and each other. Society most truly should know the value of the nurse as a healing presence, the person who, with knowledge and competence, *compassionately* and *passionately* cares and advocates for the healing and well-being of all. Begin with being compassionate to yourself and passionate about yourself. Then reconnect with others.

The most potent nursing intervention we have at our disposal is not technological in nature, nor is it directly related to our knowledge and skills. It is related more to our humanness and the ability to provide true presence, in whatever capacity we can offer it. Nurses have a responsibility, a personal and professional ethic, and the *power* to knowingly engage in health care practices that benefit *us* and *others*. We bring gifts to our community of patients every day; it is our calling to do so. Yet, as author Dan Millman (2000) notes: "if we wait until we have permission, until we feel more motivated, until it gets easier, until fear vanishes, or hell freezes over, we may miss the chance to act at all" (p. 74). Do not let a lifetime of precious moments go by. As I tell seniors getting ready to go out into the world of nursing: Robots are not wanted here!

The end result of a windfall or snowball effect is transformational change; nothing less is called for in this era where there is a critical shortage of nurses and recruitment and retention of experienced staff is an ever-increasing problem. Combined with enormous challenges in the provision of quality care related to economic burdens, it is more than time to build a community of self and other care. It is time to heal ourselves and each other.

Whether you are currently in practice or in school, look carefully at the prospects before you. Is there ample opportunity for you to round out your skills to enable you to be all that you can be? You do not need to learn more about that barnyard of chickens that Chenevert (1988) wrote about. You want to learn how to fly! Perhaps you are an eagle or perhaps you are a butterfly. . . .

> Above them were thousands and thousands of monarchs riding a current across the sky. It was impossible to guess exactly how many there were. She felt humbled watching them. These fragile, heroic voyagers, each following an age-old instinct, formed a magnificent river of purpose flowing across the sky.
>
> —*Monroe, 2011, p. 321*

Imagine. Millions of nurses all working *together in harmony*. Transformers of living-dying, engaged in the most important work there is—for what could be more important than assisting people to actualize their potentials to live well and die well? Nurses are just like butterflies, we make people smile and we transform, for the better, those whose lives we touch. We are fragile, and we are heroic. We *are* a magnificent river of purpose flowing through health care.

APPENDIX A: PROQOL VERSION 5 (STAMM, 2009–2011)

COMPASSION SATISFACTION AND COMPASSION FATIGUE
(PROQOL) VERSION 5 (2009)

When you [help] people you have direct contact with their lives. As you may have found, your compassion for those you [help] can affect you in positive and negative ways. Below are some-questions about your experiences, both positive and negative, as a [helper]. Consider each of the following questions about you and your current work situation. Select the number that honestly reflects how frequently you experienced these things in the **last 30 days.**

I=Never	2=Rarely	3=Sometimes	4=Often	5=Very Often

_____ 1. I am happy.

_____ 2. I am preoccupied with more than one person I [help].

_____ 3. I get satisfaction from being able to [help] people.

_____ 4. I feel connected to others.

_____ 5. I jump or am startled by unexpected sounds.

_____ 6. I feel invigorated after working with those I [help].

_____ 7. I find it difficult to separate my personal life from my life as a [helper].

_____ 8. I am not as productive at work because I am losing sleep over traumatic experiences of a person I [help].

_____ 9. I think that I might have been affected by the traumatic stress of those I [help].

_____ 10. I feel trapped by my job as a [helper].

_____ 11. Because of my [helping, I have felt "on edge" about various things.]

_____ 12. I like my work as a [helper].

_____ 13. I feel depressed because of the traumatic experiences of the people I [help].

_____ 14. I feel as though I am experiencing the trauma of someone I have [helped].

_____ 15. I have beliefs that sustain me.

_____ 16. I am pleased with how I am able to keep up with [helping] techniques and protocols.

_____ 17. I am the person I always wanted to be.

_____ 18. My work makes me feel satisfied.

_____ 19. I feel worn out because of my work as a [helper].

_____ 20. I have happy thoughts and feelings about those I [help] and how I could help them.

_____ 21. I feel overwhelmed because my case [work] load seems endless.

_____ 22. I believe I can make a difference through my work.

_____ 23. I avoid certain activities or situations because they remind me of frightening experiences of the people I [help].

_____ 24. I am proud of what I can do to [help].

_____ 25. As a result of my [helping], I have intrusive, frightening thoughts.

_____ 26. I feel "bogged down" by the system.

_____ 27. I have thoughts that I am a "success" as a [helper].

_____ 28. I can't recall important parts of my work with trauma victims.

_____ 29. I am a very caring person.

_____ 30. I am happy that I chose to do this work.

YOUR SCORES ON THE PROQOL: PROFESSIONAL QUALITY OF LIFE SCREENING

Based on your responses, place your personal scores below. If you have any concerns, you should discuss them with a physical or mental health care professional.

Compassion Satisfaction _____

Compassion satisfaction is about the pleasure you derive from being able to do your work well. For example, you may feel like it is a pleasure to help others through your work. You may feel positively about your colleagues or your ability to contribute to the work setting or even the greater good of society. Higher scores on this scale represent a greater satisfaction related to your ability to be an effective caregiver in your job.

The average score is 50 (SD 10; alpha scale reliability .88). About 25% of people score higher than 57 and about 25% of people score below 43. If you are in the higher range, you probably derive a good deal of professional satisfaction from your position. If your scores are below 40, you may either find problems with your job, or there may be some other reason—for example, you might derive your satisfaction from activities other than your job.

Burnout_____

Most people have an intuitive idea of what burnout is. From the research perspective, burnout is one of the elements of Compassion Fatigue (CF). It is associated with feelings of hopelessness and difficulties in dealing with work or in doing your job effectively. These negative feelings usually have a gradual onset. They can reflect the feeling that your efforts make no difference, or they can be associated with a very high workload or a non-supportive work environment. Higher scores on this scale mean that you are at higher risk for burnout.

The average score on the burnout scale is 50 (SD 10; alpha scale reliability .75). About 25% of people score above 57 and about 25% of people score below 43. If your score is below 43, this probably reflects positive feelings about your ability to be effective in your work. If you score above 57 you may wish to think about what at work makes you feel like you are not effective in your position. Your score may reflect your mood; perhaps you were having a "bad day" or are in need of some time off. If the high score persists or if it is reflective of other worries, it may be a cause for concern.

Secondary Traumatic Stress_____

The second component of Compassion Fatigue (CF) is secondary traumatic stress (STS). It is about your work related, secondary exposure to extremely or traumatically stressful events. Developing problems due to exposure to other's trauma is somewhat rare but does happen to many people who care for those who have experienced extremely or traumatically stressful events. For example, you may repeatedly hear stories about the traumatic things that happen to other people, commonly called Vicarious Traumatization. If your work puts you directly in the path of danger, for example, field work in a war or area of civil violence, this is not secondary exposure; your exposure is primary. However, if you are exposed to others' traumatic events as a result of your work, for example, as a therapist or an emergency worker, this is secondary exposure. The symptoms of STS are usually rapid in onset and associated with a particular event. They may include being afraid, having difficulty sleeping, having images of the upsetting event pop into your mind, or avoiding things that remind you of the event.

The average score on this scale is 50 (SD 10; alpha scale reliability .81). About 25% of people score below 43 and about 25% of people score above 57. If your score is above 57, you may want to take some time to think about what at work may be frightening to you or if there is some other reason for the elevated score. While higher scores do not mean that you do have a problem, they are an indication that you may want to examine how you feel about your work and your work environment. You may wish to discuss this with your supervisor, a colleague, or a health care professional.

WHAT IS MY SCORE AND WHAT DOES IT MEAN?

In this section, you will score your test and then you can compare your score to the interpretation below.

To find your score on **each section,** total the questions listed on the left in each section and then find your score in the table on the right of the section.

Compassion Satisfaction Scale:

3. _____
6. _____
12. _____
16. _____
18. _____
20. _____
22. _____
24. _____
27. _____
30. _____
Total: _____

The sum of my Compassion Satisfaction questions	So My Score Equals	My Level of Compassion
22 or less	43 or less	Low
Between 23 and 41	Around 50	Average
42 or more	57 or more	High

Burnout Scale:

*1. _____ = _____
*4. _____ = _____
8. _____
10. _____
*15. _____ = _____
*17. _____ = _____
19. _____
21. _____
26. _____
*29. _____ = _____

Reverse the scores for those that are starred.
0=0, 1=5, 2=4, 3=3, 4=2, 5=1
Total: _____

The sum of my Burnout Questions	So My Score Equals	My Level of Burnout
22 or less	43 or less	Low
Between 23 and 41	Around 50	Average
42 or more	57 or more	High

Secondary Trauma Scale:

2. _____
5. _____
7. _____
9. _____
11. _____
13. _____
14. _____
23. _____
25. _____
28. _____
Total: _____

The sum of my Secondary Traumatic Stress questions	So My Score Equals	My Level of Secondary Traumatic Stress
22 or less	43 or less	Low
Between 23 and 41	Around 50	Average
42 or more	57 or more	High

APPENDIX B: PPACD R-I (TODARO-FRANCESCHI, 2010)

Perception of Preparedness and Ability to Care for the Dying (PPACD) R-I Scale © Todaro-Franceschi

DIRECTIONS: Please circle one best answer for each question	Comments
1. I feel very comfortable listening and talking to patients and their loved ones about death, dying and bereavement. • Strongly Agree • Agree • Disagree • Strongly disagree	
2. I rate myself as highly competent in my ability to talk to patients and their loved ones about death, dying and bereavement. • Strongly Agree • Agree • Disagree • Strongly disagree	
3. Compared to your colleagues, how would you rate your competency regarding your ability to talk and listen to patients and their loved ones about death and bereavement? • Much more • More • A little less • Much less	
4. I rate myself as highly competent in my ability to provide pain and symptom management at the end of life. • Strongly agree • Agree • Disagree • Strongly disagree	
5. Compared to your colleagues, how would you rate your competency regarding your ability to provide pain and symptom management at the end of life? • Much more • More • A little less • Much less	
6. Generally speaking, do you feel able to provide quality care to the dying and their loved ones? • Yes • No	

RESOURCES

The following list is a small sample of the materials available on the internet related to topics covered herein. It is meant to be only a starting point for more information. Please note that some of these resources may fit other categories as well—it is all one!

All of these websites were accessible as we went to press. Since then, they may have changed or may no longer be available.

Healing Compassion Fatigue

Professional Quality of Life Elements Theory and Measurement: Provides extensive, free access to research and data regarding compassion satisfaction, compassion fatigue (secondary traumatic stress), and burnout. Includes Beth Stamm's "Professional Quality of Life" (ProQOL) Scale to assess compassion satisfaction, fatigue, and burnout. Additional materials can be accessed at this site, along with an extensive reference list compiled by Beth Stamm and colleagues. http://www.proqol.org

Compassion Fatigue Awareness Project: Provides information to promote awareness about compassion fatigue and its effects on carers. Offers educational workshops, suggested reading, self-tests, and other resources. http://www.compassionfatigue.org/

Compassion Fatigue Solutions: Canadian-based website—creators provide consulting services, training materials, workshops, a bookstore, blog, and events. http://compassionfatigue.ca/

Sterling Heart: Caring for Caregivers: Identifies resources for health care professionals regarding compassion fatigue, burnout, grief/loss, and stress relief through the use of readings, music, self-care tips, and workshops. Also acknowledges the importance of spirituality and provides guidance for deepening spirituality. http://www.sterlingheart.com/index.html

The Headington Institute: Care for Caregivers Worldwide: Specifically targets relief and humanitarian workers. Offers trainings, counseling, and a variety of online resources, including podcasts, self assessment questionnaires, and workshop outlines. http://www.headington-institute.org

Watson Caring Science Institute: Dr. Jean Watson is a distinguished nurse scholar, theorist, and educator. She offers insight into the caring and healing we do as nurses and encouragement to persevere through hardship. *http://www.watsoncaringscience.org/index.cfm?fuseaction=page.dis play&page_id=21*

Watson's The Caring Moment: There is a link on the above site to a poignant audio file of Jean Watson speaking about the power of a caring moment. http://www.watsoncaringscience.org/files/media/caring_moment.mp3

Companion Arts: This is a nonprofit organization dedicated to providing resources to caregivers and includes links to other influential speakers. http://www.companionarts.org/care2jean.htm

Dr. Elizabeth Barrett: Elizabeth A. M. Barrett is a distinguished nurse scholar, theorist, and practitioner. This site gives an overview of her theory of power as knowing participation in change, along with information on health patterning, power prescriptions, and the Power-Imagery Process co-developed with imagery pioneer and physician Jerry Epstein. http://www.drelizabethbarrett.com/

Commonweal: This nonprofit health and research institute aims to create a safer world for all people. More specifically, the Institute for the Study of Health & Illness offers a variety of programs for health care professionals to reconnect with compassionate healing work. http://www.commonweal.org/

Organizations Dedicated to Healing Trauma

Traumatology Institute: Dedicated to alleviating trauma through education, research, and training. This organization offers training and certification in a variety of areas related to trauma, including compassion fatigue, and also courses to become a Clinical Traumatologist and a Compassion Fatigue specialist. http://www.psychink.com/index.html

Gifts From Within: PTSD Resources for Survivors and Caregivers: DVDs, background information, an extensive collection of webcasts, art, music, poetry (for members), support groups, retreats, conferences, workshops, meditation techniques, and both humorous and inspirational stories. http://www.giftfromwithin.org/html/What-is-Compassion-Fatigue-Dr-Charles-Figley.html

The Figley Institute: This institute aims to alleviate the impact of trauma for both professionals and nonprofessionals through trauma training at various education levels. They provide online courses, workshops, and trainings. They also offer certification courses to become a Field Traumatologist, Compassion Fatigue Educator, and Certified Traumatologist. http://www.figleyinstitute.com/

The Sidran Institute: Traumatic Stress Education and Advocacy—The philosophy of this institute is to help heal trauma through connection and empowerment. They offer an extensive resource list to promote education and self-help, which includes books, workbooks, textbooks, training manuals, DVDs and videos, and educational tools. They also have ongoing projects nationwide, education programming, and trainings. http://www.sidran.org/

Traumatic Incident Reduction Association: Traumatic Incident Reduction Therapy is a method used to reduce stress associated with past traumatic experiences. The website offers links to professionals, trainings, and workshops to help cope with and overcome trauma (includes a recovery program specific to compassion fatigue). http://www.tir.org/research_pub/research/compassion_fatigue.html

The Green Cross: This traumatology academy offers support and guidance in times of acute crisis or trauma through crisis counseling, ongoing counseling, and referral services. Additionally, this institute contains training programs to become a certified Traumatologist or Compassion Fatigue Educator/Therapist. http://greencross.org/

Bullying Resources

Life After Bullying: This website offers a general overview of bullying (what it is, who does it, who are the targets), as well as self-help tips, explanation of employer liability, links to finding counseling, as well as links to articles and other resources. http://www.lifeafteradultbullying.com/index.html

The Workplace Bullying Institute: The goal of this organization is to understand and prevent workplace abuse. The website is very extensive and offers a wealth of information about bullying, emphasizing that the victim is not alone and not helpless. Resources include access to research and legislation, a blog, training for individuals, professionals, and employers, coaching and the creation of an action plan for individuals being bullied, speeches, books, audio recordings, and DVDs. http://www.workplacebullying.org/

American Nurses Association: The organization website offers an abundance of resource materials for nurses, including information on workplace violence and safety. http://www.nursingworld.org/MainMenuCategories/WorkplaceSafety/workplaceviolence

Center for American Nurses: A fact sheet and free webinars on workplace bullying are available. The position statement on lateral violence is accessible here as well as tip cards, webinars, literature, videos, and additional resources. The pdfs of the tip cards can be downloaded for free. http://www.can.affiniscape.com/displaycommon.cfm?an=1&subarticlenbr =283

Juice in Healthcare: This organization promotes positive energy in the workplace. The website offers general resources for overcoming a negative or hostile work environment, such as articles, e-books, videos, case studies as well as some specific to nurse-to-nurse hostility (some are for purchase only). http://www.juiceinc.com/about/healthcare

Healing Addiction Resources

Addiction Recovery Resources for the Professional: Includes information on addiction and recovery, self-test, book list and resources list, stories, and support for finding help. http://www.lapage.com/arr/

Hazelden: This organization specializes in addiction treatment and has a specific program for health care professionals. The program includes group therapy, tips for reentry into the workplace, lectures, and peer-to-peer support. http://www.hazelden.org/web/public/addiction_treatment_health_care_professionals.page

Unbecoming a Nurse: Bypassing the Hidden Chemical Dependency Trap: This website was developed by nurse Paula Davies Scimeca and is a supplement for her authored book on the subject, to offer help for nurses struggling with substance abuse. The website has a variety of resources including FAQs, interviews, a blog, articles, events, retreats, a self-survey, and a list of other resources. http://www.unbecominganurse.org/

NurseNRecovery: Designed to provide help and hope for nurses suffering from addiction, the website has forums and information/links for treatment options. http://www.nursenrecovery.com

Peer Advocacy for Impaired Nurses: Founded by Jack Stem, a recovering CRNA, this website offers a wealth of information and resourceful links. He also offers educational workshops, recovery mentoring, and relapse prevention to individual nurses. http://www.peeradvocacyforimpaired nurses.com

The Addiction Recovery Guide: Extensive guide to help with addiction recovery for anyone suffering with substance abuse/addiction. Includes links to programs nationwide, a message board, alternative therapies, and relapse prevention resources. http://www.addictionrecoveryguide.org/

On Mindfulness

Mindful: All about being mindful—"living with awareness and compassion." Created by Shambhala Sun Foundation. http://www.mindful.org/

Mindful Hub: Wellbeing, Right Now: This website is dedicated to encouraging healthcare professionals to practice being mindful and also has specific information regarding compassion fatigue. It offers free worksheets and newsletters, articles, resources, and e-consultation (for a fee). http://mindfulhub.com/archives/2011/08/combating-compassion-fatigue-with-mindfulness/

Stress Relief Choices: This website addresses stress relief for healthcare professionals and offers tips such as including exercise and healthy eating as well as meditation, deep breathing, and visualization. Coaching, classes, as well as free resources, a newsletter, and recommended reading is also available. http://www.stress-relief-choices.com/stress-management-for-nurses.html

American Holistic Nurses Association: Their website offers information and techniques for stress management, including, yoga, tai chi, dance, art, massage, journaling, energy work, and prayer. http://www.ahna.org/Resources/StressManagement/ManagingStress/tabid/1813/Default.aspx

Resources on Assertiveness

Livestrong: The Limitless Potential of You: This website outlines what assertive behavior is and addresses myths and rights regarding assertiveness. http://www.livestrong.com/article/14699-improving-assertive-behavior/

Assertiveness Quiz—This quiz evaluates one's level of assertiveness and offers links to articles regarding conflict resolution and communication, including benefits of assertiveness, daily stress tips, and how to improve relationships. http://stress.about.com/library/assertiveness_quiz/bl_assertiveness_quiz.htm

Skills Converged: Training Materials on Productivity, Soft Skills, and Personal Development: This website offers free training resources, games, icebreakers, role-plays and exercises regarding team building, time management, communication skills, conflict resolution, and emotional intelligence for all ages and groups. My favorite: *The Butterfly Effect,* an exercise that demonstrates how a subtle change can have a lasting and far-reaching impact. http://www.skillsconverged.com/Home/tabid/229/Default.aspx

Moral Distress and Help With Ethical Dilemmas

American Nurses Association: Link to our code of ethics, position statements, and a number of excellent online journal articles related to moral distress and moral courage. http://www.nursingworld.org/MainMenuCategories/EthicsStandards/CodeofEthicsforNurses

American Association of Critical Care Nurses (AACN) Ask Affirm Assess Act: The 4 A's to Rise Above Moral Distress is a wonderful guide to help nurses recognize and address moral distress in the work place. http://www.aacn.org/WD/Practice/Docs/4As_to_Rise_Above_Moral_Distress.pdf

AACN also offers a free Healthy Work Environment Assessment Tool: http://www.hweteamtool.org/main/index

All About Compassion and Healthy Work Environments

Center for Building a Culture of Empathy: Dedicated to building a worldwide community of compassion and empathy. Includes articles, conferences, definitions, expert opinions, historical and scientific information, interviews, and videos. http://cultureofempathy.com

Empathy and Healthcare: (from the above website) A collection of articles from the news about empathy and healthcare. http://www.scoop. it/t/empathy-and-healthcare/

Compassion Lab: This organization is made up of a collection of researchers offering resources to enable the creation of organizations using a compassionate foundation. The website includes teaching materials, presentations, publications, and access to like-minded researchers. http://www.compassionlab.com/

TED Conferences: A collection of inspirational speeches and talks regarding compassion. http://www.ted.com/themes/the_charter_for_compassion.html

Positive Psychology: This website is dedicated to promoting positivity and happiness, in thought and action. There is access to literature, related resources, and an annual conference. http://www.positivepsychology.net/

The Center for Nonviolent Communication: This international organization is founded on the basis that we are all compassionate, nonviolent beings. Through trainings, video, audio, resources, bookstore, e-forums, connection to others, and more, they encourage embracing a nonviolent ideology to resolve conflict peacefully and effectively. http://www.cnvc.org/

Passion Works! Creating Passion in the Workplace—Started by a group of development professionals, this website is dedicated to helping leaders and individuals generate passion in the workplace. The site includes access to research, literature, diagnostic tools, coaching services, conferences, and workshops. http://www.passionworks.com/en/home/default.aspx

AACN's Healthy Work Environments Initiative: Promotes healthy work environments through conferences, continuing education, research, and collaboration. http://www.aacn.org/wd/hwe/content/hwehome.pcms?menu=hwe

Heartmath: Aims to promote health and well being through training programs, publications, and "emWave" technology, resulting in outcomes including: employee retention, reduced costs, decreased stress and anxiety, and increased productivity. Contains a section specific to health care. http://www.heartmath.com/

Center for Positive Organizational Scholarship: Dedicated to improving leadership through "positive organizing." The website offers a wide array of substantial resources, including suggestions for beginners, education opportunities, literature, teaching materials, and video. http://www.centerforpos.org/

Project Resilience: Through trainings, information, and teaching materials, this organization supports administrators and supervisors in creating a more supportive work environment, particularly in regards to overcoming hardships, such as addiction or violence. http://projectresilience.com/index.htm

Information on Burnout

European Institute for Intervention and Research on Burnout: This website includes information, self-test, news, coping techniques, trainings, and seminars. http://www.burnout-institute.org/index_en.php

Headington Institute: Provides a description of burnout, ways to protect yourself against burnout, and various self-tests. http://www.headington-institute.org/Default.aspx?tabid=1791

Center for Professional Wellbeing: Offers information and coping techniques to deal with burnout as well as consultation, trainings, and suggested reading. http://www.cpwb.org/burnout_information.htm

Information on End-of-Life Care (and Education)

American Association of Colleges in Nursing ELNEC: ELNEC program information is available through their website along with a frequently updated list of ELNEC program offerings. There is also a link to web resources related to end-of-life care. http://www.aacn.nche.edu/elnec

City of Hope Pain and Palliative Care Resource Center: Their website offers a database of reference materials regarding end-of-life care, along with an extensive web-based listing of other internet websites. http://prc.coh.org/

Hospice and Palliative Nurses Association: This organization is dedicated to promoting excellence in hospice and palliative nursing care. The website offers information on education and resources for nurses. http://www.hpna.org

National Hospice and Palliative Care Organization (NHPCO): Dedicated to improving the quality of care at the end of life through hospice and palliative care efforts. A wealth of materials. http://www.nhpco.org/templates/1/homepage.cfm

National Hospice Foundation: A partner organization of NHPCO, their website offers additional information on end-of-life care. http://www.nationalhospicefoundation.org/home.cfm

Center to Advance Palliative Care: Offers materials to aid in development of palliative care programs. Palliative care tools, education, resources, and training for health care professionals can be accessed through their site. http://www.capc.org/

Hastings Center: This organization is dedicated to addressing, through research, education, and policy-making, ethical issues in health, medicine, and the environment that affect people. A significant part of their work deals with end-of-life care. http://www.thehastingscenter.org/Issues/Default.aspx?v=244

On Appreciative Inquiry

Appreciative Inquiry Commons: Dedicated to the study, application and dissemination of information related to appreciative inquiry. They offer many resources, including access to classic articles and case exemplars. http://appreciativeinquiry.case.edu/

To See Things You Normally Do Not See

The Energy Enigma: My website on the enigma of energy, death and dying, and synchronicity. www.energy-enigma.com

Journey North: On this website you can sign up to receive e-news on the migration of various wildlife—monarchs, hummingbirds, whooping cranes, and lots of other signs of spring news. You can also report your sightings. http://journeynorth.org/

Monarch Watch: For more information on the monarch butterfly and the migration. www.monarchwatch.org

To follow my work on this subject:

Quality Caring: A website for nurses and other health care professionals interested in enhancing quality caring for both the cared for and the carers. Blog, links, and other resources. www.qualitycaring.org

All of the opinions and information on these websites is theirs, not mine. I have no investment or interest (other than my own website). Readers should make note of individual website policies regarding privacy and membership. Every website differs.

REFERENCES

Aiken, L., Clarke, S., Sloane, D., & Sochalski, J. (2001). An international perspective on hospital nurse's work environments: The case for reform. *Policy, Politics, and Nursing Practice, 2*, 255–263.

Aiken, L., Clarke, S., Sloane, D., Sochalski, J., & Silber, J. (2002). Hospital nurse staffing and patient mortality, nurse burnout and job dissatisfaction. *Journal of the American Medical Association, 288*(16), 1987–1993.

Aiken, L. H., Sloane, D. M., Clarke, S., Poghosyan, L., Cho, E., You, L. et al. (2011). Importance of work environments on hospital outcomes in nine countries. *International Journal for Quality in Health Care, 23*(4) 357–364.

Albom, M. (1997). *Tuesdays with Morrie: An old man, a young man, and life's greatest lesson.* New York: Doubleday.

American Association of Colleges in Nursing (AACN) & City of Hope National Medical Center (COH). (1999). *End of life nursing education consortium project (ELNEC).* Washington, DC: Authors.

American Association of Critical Care Nurses Ethics Work Group. (2006). *The 4 A's to rise above moral distress.* Retrieved from http://www.aacn.org/WD/Practice/Docs/4As_to_Rise_Above_Moral_Distress.pdf

American Nurses Credentialing Center (ANCC). (2008). *Application manual: Magnet recognition program.* Silver Spring, MD: Author.

Angeles, P. A. (1992). *The Harper Collins dictionary of philosophy* (2nd ed.). New York: Harper Perennial.

Angus, D. C., Barnato, A. E., Linde-Zwirble, W. T., Weissfeld, L. A., Watson, R. S., Rickert, T., Rickert, T., Rubenfeld, G. D., & Robert Wood Johnson Foundation ICU End-Of-Life Peer Group. (2004). Use of intensive care at the end of life in the United States: An epidemiologic study. *Critical Care Medicine, 32*(3), 638–643.

Anticau, K. (2008). *Ruby's imagine.* Boston: Houghton Mifflin Company.

Aristotle. (n.d./1984). *The complete works of Aristotle: The revised Oxford translation* (Vol. 1–2), J. Barnes, (Ed.) Princeton, NJ: Princeton University Press.

Aristotle. (n.d./1911). *The Nichomachean ethics* (D. P. Chase, Trans.). London: J. M. Dent & Sons Ltd.

Aristotle. (n.d./1991). *The metaphysics* (J. H. McMahon, Trans.). Buffalo, NY: Prometheus Books.

Aristotle. (n.d./1996). *Physics* (R. Waterfield, Trans.). New York: Oxford University Press.

Auden, W. H. (1940). *Another time.* New York: Random House.

Balducci, D. (2000). *Wish you well.* New York: Warner Books.

Barnes, J. (1982). *Aristotle.* New York: Oxford University Press.

Barrett, E. A. M. (1989). A nursing theory of power for nursing practice. In J. P. Riehl-Sisca (Ed.), *Conceptual models for nursing practice* (3rd ed., pp. 207–217). Norwalk, CT: Appleton & Lange.

Barrett, E. A. M. (2010). Power as knowing participation in change: What's new and what's next. *Nursing Science Quarterly, 23*(1), 47–54.

Baumrucker, S. J. (2002). Palliative care, burnout, and the pursuit of happiness. *American Journal of Hospice and Palliative Care, 19,* 154–156.

Belitz, C., & Lundstrom, M. (1997). *The power of flow: Practical ways to transform your life with meaningful coincidence.* New York: Harmony Books.

Benner, P. (1984). *From novice to expert: Excellence and power in clinical nursing practice.* Menlo Park, CA: Addison-Wesley Publishing.

Benner, P. (1994). Caring as a way of knowing and not knowing. In S. S. Phillips & P. Benner (Eds.). *The crisis of care: Affirming and restoring caring practices in the helping professions* (pp. 42–62). Washington, DC: Georgetown University Press.

Benner, P., Sutphen, M., Leonard, V., Day, L., & Shulman, L. [Foreword]. (2009). *Educating nurses: A call for radical transformation* (Jossey-Bass/Carnegie Foundation for the Advancement of Teaching). Kindle Edition. Retrieved from www.amazon.com

Benoliel, J. Q. (1973). The practitioner's dilemma: Problems and priorities. In J. Q. Benoliel, H. Feifel, E. S. Shneidman, C. W. Wahl, & E. H. Waechter (Eds.), *Dealing with death* (pp. 33–45). Los Angeles, CA: University of Southern California.

Benson, J., & Magraith, K. (2005). Compassion fatigue and burnout: The role of Balint groups. *Australian Family Physician, 34*(6), 497–498.

Bilgel, N., Aytac, S., & Bayram, N. (2006). Bullying in Turkish white-collar workers. *Occupational Medicine, 56,* 226–231.

Billings, M. E., Engelberg, R., Curtis, J. R., Block, S., & Sullivan, A. M. (2010). Determinants of medical students' perceived preparation to perform end of life care, quality of end of life care education, and attitudes toward end of life care. *Journal of Palliative Medicine, 13*(3), 319–326.

Bishop, A. H., & Scudder, J. R. (1996). *Nursing ethics: Therapeutic caring presence.* Sudbury, MA: Jones and Bartlett.

Blum, L. Compassion. (1980). In A. M. Rorty (Ed.). *Explaining emotions* (pp. 507–517). Berkeley, CA: University of California Press.

Böckerman, P., & Ilmakunnas, P. (2008). Interaction of working conditions, job satisfaction, and sickness absences: Evidence from a representative sample of employees. *Soc Sci Med. 67*(4), 520–528.

Bohm, D. (1996). *On dialogue.* London: Routledge.

Bohm, D. (1998). In L. Nichol (Ed.), *On creativity.* New York: Routledge.

Briggs, J., & Peat, D. (1999). *Seven life lessons of chaos: Spiritual wisdom from the science of change.* New York: HarperCollins.

Broome, B. A., & Williams-Evans, S. (2011). Bullying in a caring profession: Reasons, results and recommendations. *Journal of Psychosocial Nursing, 49,* 30–35.

Buerhaus, P. I. (2008). Current and future state of the U.S. nursing workforce. *Journal of the American Medical Association, 300*(20), 2422–2424.

Burnell, L. (2009). Compassionate care: A concept analysis. *Home Health Care Management and Practice, 21,* 319–324.

Callahan, D. (1991). Medical futility, medical necessity: The problem-without-a-name. *Hastings Center Report, 21*(4), 30–35.

Capra, F., Steindl-Rast, D., & Matus, T. (1991). *Belonging to the universe: Explorations on the frontiers of science and spirituality.* San Francisco, CA: Harper & Row.

Carper, B. A. (1978). Fundamental patterns of knowing in nursing. *Advances in Nursing Science, 1*(1), 13–24.

Cassell, E. J. (2005). Chapter 31: Compassion. In C. R. Snyder, & S. J. Lopez (Eds.), *Handbook of positive psychology* (pp. 434–445). Cary, NC: Oxford University Press.

Center for American Nurses. (2008). *Lateral violence and bullying in the workplace.* Retrieved from http://www.centerforamericannurses.org/associations/9102/files/position%20statementlateral%20violence%20and%20bullying.pdf

Center to Advance Palliative Care and the National Palliative Care Research Center. (2008). *America's care of serious illness: A state-by-state report card on access to palliative care in our nation's hospitals.* Retrieved from http://www.capc.org/reportcard

Chenevert, M. (1985). *Pro-nurse handbook: Designed for the nurse who wants to survive/thrive professionally.* St. Louis: C.V. Mosby.

Chenevert, M. (1988). *STAT: Special techniques in assertiveness training for women in the health professions.* St. Louis, MO: C.V. Mosby.

Chodron, P. (2001). *The places that scare you: A guide to fearlessness in difficult times.* Boston, MA: Shambala.

City of Hope (COH) and American Association of Colleges in Nursing (AACN). (2011). *ELNEC core curriculum.* Washington, DC: Authors.

Clark, C. (2010, 3/21/10). Why civility matters. *Sigma Theta Tau International Reflections on Leadership, 36*(1). Retrieved from http://www.reflectionsonnursingleadership.com/pages/vol36_1_clark2_civility.aspx

Clark, C., & Farnsworth, J. (2006). Program for recovering nurses: An evaluation. *Medsurg Nursing, 15*(4), 223–224.

Clayton, G. M., Murray, J. P., Horner, S. D., & Greene, P. E. (1991). Chapter 12. Connecting: A catalyst for caring. In P. L. Chinn (Ed.), *Anthology on caring* (pp. 155–168). New York: National League for Nursing.

Cleary, M., Hunt, G. E., & Horsfall, J. (2010). Identifying and addressing bullying in nursing. *Issues in Mental Health Nursing, 31*, 331–335.

Cleveland Clinic. (2011, Spring). Nurse researchers examine relationships and bullying in the workplace. *Notable Nursing, 13.* Accessed at http://my.clevelandclinic.org/Documents/nursing/notableNursingSpring2011.pdf

Conant, E. (2007, March 19). To share in the horror. *Newsweek, 149*(12), 34.

Cooperrider, D. L., & Whitney, D. (2005). *Appreciative inquiry: A positive revolution in change.* San Francisco: Berrett-Koehler Publishers.

Corley, M. C. (2002). Nurse moral distress: A proposed theory and research agenda. *Nursing Ethics, 9*(6), 636–650.

Coyle, N. (2006). The hard work of living in the face of death. *Journal of Pain and Symptom Management, 32*(3), 266–274.

Csikszentmihalyi, M. (1990). *Flow: The psychology of optimal experience.* New York: Harper & Row.

Dalai Lama & Cutler, H. C. (1998). *The art of happiness: A handbook for living.* New York: Riverhead Books.

Davies, E. (2004). *What are the palliative care needs of older people and how might they be met? A health evidence network synthesis report.* World Health Organization: Regional Office for Europe. Retrieved from http://www.euro.who.int/HEN/Syntheses/palliative/20040722_

Djukic, M., Kovner, C. T., Brewer, C. S., Fatehi, F. K., & Cline, D. D. (2011). Nurse work environment factors other than staffing associated with nurses' ratings of patient care quality. *Health Care Management Review.* Advance online publication. Retrieved from http://rnworkproject.org/resource_type/published-paper/

Dossey, L. (2007). Compassion. *Explorations, 3*(1), 1–5.

Drenkard, K., Wolf, G., & Morgan, S. H. (Eds.). (2011). *Magnet: The next generation-nurses making the difference*. Silver Spring, MD: American Nurses Credentialing Center.

Dutton, J. E., Frost, P. J., Worline, M. C., Lilius, J. M., & Kanov, J. M. (2002). Leading in times of trauma. *Harvard Business Review, 80*(1), 54–61.

Edmonson, C. (2010). Moral courage and the nurse leader. *The Online Journal of Issues in Nursing, 15*(3), Manuscript 5. Accessed at http://www.nursing world.org/MainMenuCategories/ANAMarketplace/ANAPeriodicals/ OJIN/TableofContents/Vol152010/No3-Sept-2010/Moral-Courage-for-Nurse-Leaders.html

Einstein, A. (1954). *Ideas and opinions*. New York: Wings Books.

Erikson, K. T. (1995). Loss of communality at Buffalo Creek. In J. B. Williamson, & E. S. Slimeidman (Eds.), *Death: Current perspectives* (4th ed., pp. 407–413). Mountain View, CA: Mayfield Publishing.

Fawcett, J. (2005). *Contemporary nursing knowledge: Analysis and evaluation of nursing models and theories* (2nd ed.). Philadelphia, PA: F. A. Davis.

Ferrell, B. (2006). Understanding the moral distress of nurses witnessing medically futile care. *Oncology Nursing Forum, 33*, 922–930.

Ferrell, B., & Coyle, N. (2008). *The nature of suffering and the goals of nursing*. New York: Oxford University Press.

Figley, C. R. (1995). *Compassion fatigue: Coping with secondary traumatic stress disorder in those who treat the traumatized*. New York: Brunner Mazel.

Figley, C. R. (2002a). Compassion fatigue: Psychotherapists' chronic lack of self care. *Journal of Clinical Psychology, 58*(11), 1433–1441.

Figley, C. R. (Ed.). (2002b). *Treating compassion fatigue*. New York: Brunner-Routledge.

Finkelman, A., & Kenner, C. (2009). *Teaching IOM: Implications of the Institute of Medicine reports for nursing education* (2nd ed.). Silver Spring, MD: American Nurses Association.

Forster, D. (2009). Rethinking compassion fatigue as moral distress. *Journal of Ethics in Mental Health, 4*, 1–4.

Fowler, M. D. M. (Ed.). (2008). *Guide to the code of ethics for nurses: Interpretation and application*. Silver Spring, MD: American Nurses Association.

Frankl, V. (1959). *Man's search for meaning*. New York: Beacon Press.

Freudenberger, H. J. (1975). The staff burnout syndrome in alternative institutions. *Psychotherapy, Theory, Research and Practice, 12*, 72–83.

Freudenberger, H. J., & North, G. (1985). *Women's burnout: How to spot it, how to reverse it, and how to prevent it*. Garden City, NY: Doubleday & Company.

Frost, P. J. (1999a). Why compassion counts. *Journal of Management Inquiry, 8*(2), 127–133.

Frost, P. J. (1999b). *Toxic emotions at work and what you can do about them.* Boston: Harvard Business School Press.

Frost, P. J., Dutton, J. E., Maitlis, S., Lilius, J. M., Kanov, J. M., & Worline, M. C. (2006). Seeing organizations differently: Three lenses on compassion. In C. Hardy, S. Clegg, T. Lawrence, & W. Nord (Eds.), *Handbook of organization studies* (2nd ed., pp. 843–866). London: Sage.

Frost, P., & Robinson, S. (1999, July/August). *The toxic handler: Organizational hero—and casualty. Harvard Business Review,* 96–106.

Ganske, K. M. (2010). Moral distress in academia. *The Online Journal of Issues in Nursing, 15*(3), Manuscript. Accessed at http://www.nursingworld.org/MainMenuCategories/ANAMarketplace/ANAPeriodicals/OJIN/TableofContents/Vol152010/No3-Sept-2010/Moral-Distress-in-Academia.html

Gilligan, C. (1982). *In a different voice: Psychological theory and women's development.* Cambridge, MA: Harvard University Press.

Gladwell, M. (2000). *The tipping point: How little things can make a big difference.* New York: Little Brown.

Goldstein, K. (1963). *The organism: A holistic approach to biology derived from pathological data in man.* Boston: Beacon Press.

Goodman, D. C., Fisher, E. S., Chang, C. H., Morden, N. E., Jacobson, J. O., Murray, K., & Miesfeldt, S. (2010). *Quality of end-of-life cancer care for Medicare beneficiaries: Regional and hospital-specific analyses.* Lebanon, NH: The Dartmouth Institute.

Gordon, S. (2005). *Nursing against the odds: How health care cost cutting, media stereotypes, and medical hubris undermine nurses and patient care.* Ithaca, NY: ILR Press (an imprint of Cornell University Press).

Governance Institute. (2009). *Leadership in healthcare organizations: A guide to Joint Commission leadership standards.* Retrieved from http://www.jointcommission.org/assets/1/18/WP_leadership_standards.pdf

Greene, G. (1960). *A burnt-out case.* New York: Viking Press.

Greenwood, E. (1982). Attributes of a profession. In B. Baumrin, & B. Freedman (Eds.), *Moral responsibility and the professions* (pp. 20–32). New York: Haven Publications.

Hand, L. (2011). One fourth of ICU clinicians report inappropriate care. Accessed at http://www.medscape.com/viewarticle/756089_print

Heilburn, C. (1988). *Writing a woman's life.* New York: Ballantine Books.

Hilfiker, D. (1985). *Healing the wounds: A physician looks at his work.* New York: Pantheon Books.

Hines, D. R. (1992). Presence: Discovering the artistry in relating. *Journal of Holistic Nursing, 10*(4), 294–305.

Hooper, C., Craig, J., Janvrin, D. R., Wetsel, M. A., & Reimels, E. (2010). Compassion satisfaction, burnout, and compassion fatigue among emergency nurses compared with nurses in other selected inpatient specialties. *Journal of Emergency Nursing, 36*(5), 420–427.

Institute of Medicine (IOM). (1997). *Approaching Death: Improving care at the end of life.* Washington, DC: Author.

Institute of Medicine. (2009). Robert Wood Johnson Initiative on the Future of Nursing, at the Institute of Medicine: The future of nursing: Leading change, advancing health. National Academy of Sciences. Retrieved from http://www.iom.edu/Reports/2010/The-Future-of-Nursing-Leading-Change-Advancing-Health.aspx

James, W. (1987). *William James writings 1902–1910.* New York: The Library of America. Original work published in 1907.

Jameton, A. (1984). *Nursing practice: The ethical issues.* Englewood Cliffs, NJ: Prentice-Hall.

Jameton, A. (1993). Dilemmas of moral distress: Moral responsibility and nursing practice. *AWHONNS Clinical Issues in Perinatal & Womens Health Nursing, 4*(4), 542–551.

Johns, C. (1995). Framing learning through reflection within Carper's fundamental ways of knowing. *Journal of Advanced Nursing, 22,* 226–234.

Joinson, C. (1992). Coping with compassion fatigue. *Nursing, 22,* 116–121.

Joint Commission. (2008). *Sentinel event alert: Behaviors that undermine a culture of safety.* Retrieved from http://www.jointcommission.org/assets/1/18/SEA_40.pdf

Joint Commission. (2011). *Speak up.* Retrieved from Joint Commission: http://www.jointcommission.org/assets/1/6/speakup.pdf

Jones, J. M. (2011). *Gallup record 64% rate honesty, ethics of members of Congress low: Ratings of nurses, pharmacists, and medical doctors most positive.* Retrieved from http://www.gallup.com/poll/151460/Record-Rate-Honesty-Ethics-Members-Congress-Low.aspx

Jung, C. (1973). *Synchronicity: An acausal connecting principle* (R. F. C. Hull, Trans.). Princeton, NJ: Princeton University Press.

Kabat-Zinn, J. (1994). *Wherever you go there you are: Mindfulness meditation in everyday life.* New York: Hyperion.

Kenner, C., Finkelman, A., Weatherby, F., Long, L. E., & Kupperschmidt, B. R. (2009). Appendix K: Nursing against whose odds? Commentary on Gordon (2005) an example of teaching to the IOM reports. In A. Finkelman, & C. Kenner (Eds.), *Teaching IOM: Implications of the Institute of Medicine reports for nursing education* (2nd ed., pp. 247–256). Silver Spring, MD: American Nurses Association.

Kent, K. M. (2003). *Do it anyway: The handbook for finding personal meaning and deep happiness in a crazy world.* Maui, HI: Inner Ocean.

Ko-i Bastis, M. (2000). *Peaceful dwelling: Meditations for healing and living.* Boston, MA: Tuttle Publishing.

Kobat-Zinn, J. (1994). *Wherever you go, there you are: Mindfulness meditation in everyday life.* New York: Hyperion.

Koloroutis, M. (Ed.). (2004). *Relationship-based care: A model for transforming practice.* Minneapolis, MN: Creative Health Care Management.

Kraft, U. (2006, June/July). Burned out. *Scientific American Mind, 29*–33. Retrieved from http://www.jb-schnittstelle.de/wer/ulrich_kraft/Burned%20Out.pdf

Kubler-Ross, E. (1969). *On death and dying.* New York: Simon & Schuster.

Langle, A. (2003). Burnout—Existential meaning and possibilities of prevention. *European Psychotherapy, 4,* 107–121.

Last Acts. (2002). *Means to a better end: A report on dying in America today.* Washington, DC: Author.

Leininger, M. (Ed.). (1984). *Care: The essence of nursing and health.* Detroit, MI: Wayne State University Press.

Leininger, M. (1994). *Transcultural nursing: Concepts, theories and practices.* New York: McGraw-Hill.

Leiter, M., & Maslach, C. (2009). Nurse turnover: The mediating role of burnout. *Journal of Nursing Management, 17,* 331–339.

Levine, M. (1972). Benoni. In M. H. Browning & E. P. Lewis (Eds.), *The dying patient: A nursing perspective* (pp. 134–138). New York: The American Journal of Nursing Company.

Liaschenko, J. (2008). "... to take one's place ... and the right to have one's part matter" In W. J. E. Pinch, & A. M. Haddad (Eds.), *Nursing and health care ethics: A legacy and a vision* (pp. 195–203). Silver Spring, MD: American Nurses Association.

Liu, E., & Noppe-Brandon, S. (2009). *Imagination first: Unlocking the power of possibility.* Kindle version. San Francisco, CA: Jossey-Bass.

Longo, J. (2007). Horizontal violence among nursing students. *Archives of Psychiatric Nursing, 21,* 177–178.

Lorenz, E. (1993). *The essence of chaos.* Seattle, WA: University of Washington Press.

MacLaine, S. (2011). *I'm all over that and other confessions.* New York: Atria Books.

Magill, K. A. (1982). Burnin, burnout and the brightly burning. *Nursing Management*, *13*, 17–21.

Maisel, E. (2005). *Coaching the artist within*. Novato, CA: New World Library.

Malinski, V. M., & Barrett, E. A. M. (1994). *Martha E. Rogers: Her life and her work*. Philadelphia, PA: F. A. Davis.

Markova, D. (2000). *I will not die an unlived life: Reclaiming purpose and passion*. San Francisco, CA: Conari Press.

Maslach, C. (1976). Burned-out. *Human Behavior*, *5*, 16–22.

Maslach, C. (1982). *Burnout: The cost of caring*. Englewood Cliffs, NJ: Prentice-Hall.

Maslach, C. (1993). Burnout: A multidimensional perspective. In W. B. Schaufeli, C. Maslach, & T. Marek (Eds.), *Professional burnout: Recent developments in theory and research* (pp. 19–32). Washington, DC: Taylor & Francis.

Maslach, C., Jackson, S. E., & Leiter, M. P. (1997). Maslach burnout inventory. In: C. P. Zalaquett & R. J. Wood (Eds.), *Evaluating stress: A book of resources* (3rd ed., pp. 191–218). Lanham, MD: The Scarecrow Press, Inc.

Maslach, C., & Leiter, M. P. (1999). Take this job and love it! Six ways to beat burnout. *Psychology Today*, *32*(5), 50–53.

Maslach, C., Schaufeli, W. B., & Leiter, M. P. (2001). Job burnout. *Annual Review Psychology*, *52*, 397–422.

Maslow, A. H. (1968). *Toward a psychology of being*. New York: Van Nostrand Reinhold Co.

Maslow, A. H. (1971). *The farther reaches of human nature*. New York: The Viking Press.

Mason, D. (1999). Dancing with wolves. *American Journal of Nursing*, *99*(8), 8.

McClure, M. L. (2011). The first generation. In K. Drenkard, G. Wolf, & S. H. Morgan (Eds.), *Magnet: The next generation-nurses making the difference* (pp. 1–8). Silver Spring, MD: American Nurses Credentialing Center.

McKenna, B. G., Smith, N. A., Poole, S. J., & Coverdale, J. H. (2003). Horizontal violence: Experiences of registered nurses in their first year of practice. *Journal of Advanced Nursing*, *42*, 90–93.

Meltzer, L. S., & Huckabay, L. M. (2004). Critical care nurses' perceptions of futile care and its effect on burnout. *American Journal of Critical Care*, *13*(3), 202–207.

Millman, D. (2000). *Living on purpose: Straight answers to life's tough questions*. Novato, CA: New World Library.

Monroe, M. A. (2011). *The butterfly's daughter*. New York: Gallery Books.

Murphy, F., Jones, S., Edwards, M., James, J., & Mayer, A. (2009). The impact of nurse education on the caring behaviours of nursing students. *Nurse Education Today, 29*, 254–264.

Myss, C. (1996). *Anatomy of the spirit: The seven stages of power and healing.* New York: Harmony Books.

Newman, M. (2008). *Transforming presence: The difference that nursing makes.* Philadelphia: F. A. Davis.

Nightingale, F. (1946). *Notes on nursing: What it is, and what it is not.* (Facsimile of 1st ed.). London: Harrison and Sons. (Original work published 1859)

Nussbaum, M. (1996). Compassion: The basic social emotion. *Social Philosophy and Policy, 13*, 27–58.

Nussbaum, M. (2001). *Upheavals of thought: The intelligence of emotions.* Cambridge: Cambridge University Press.

Parker, M. E., & Smith, M. C. (2010). *Nursing theories and nursing practice* (3rd ed.). Philadelphia, PA.: F A Davis.

Parse, R. R. (1994). Quality of life: Sciencing and living the art of human becoming. *Nursing Science Quarterly, 7*, 16–21.

Parse, R. R. (1998). *The human becoming school of thought.* Thousand Oaks, CA: Sage.

Parse, R. R. (2007). The human becoming school of thought in 2050. *Nursing Science Quarterly, 20*, 308–311.

Peat, F. D. (1987). *Synchronicity: The bridge between matter and mind.* New York: Bantam.

Pereira, S. M., Fonseca, A. M., & Carvalho, A. S. (2011). Burnout in palliative care: A systematic review. *Nursing Ethics, 18*, 317–326.

Perry, B. (2008). Why exemplary oncology nurses seem to avoid compassion fatigue. *Canadian Oncology Nursing Journal, 18*(2), 87–92.

Peterson, E. H. (1994). Teaching us to care and not to care. In S. S. Phillips, & P. Benner (Eds.) *The crisis of care: Affirming and restoring caring practices in the helping professions* (pp. 66–79). Washington, DC: Georgetown University Press.

Pettigrew, J. (1990). Intensive nursing care: The ministry of presence. *Critical Care Nursing Clinics of North America, 2*, 503–508.

Pfifferling, J. H., & Gilley, K. (2000). Overcoming compassion fatigue. *Family Practice Management, 7*(4), 39–44.

Poulin, M. J., Silver, R. C., Gil-Rivas, V., Holman, E. A., & McIntosh, D. N. (2009). Finding social benefits after a collective trauma: Perceiving societal changes and well-being following 9/11. *Journal of Traumatic Stress, 22*(2), 81–90.

Prigogine, I. (1980). *From being to becoming: Time and complexity in the physical sciences*. San Francisco: Freeman.

Pross, C. (2006). Burnout, vicarious traumatization and its prevention. *Torture, 16*(1), 1–9.

Ramer, L. M. (2008). Using servant leadership to facilitate healing after a drug diversion experience. *AORN, 88*(2), 253–258.

Ramos, M. C. (2006). Eliminate destructive behaviors through example and evidence. *Nursing Management, 37*(9), 34–41.

Redfield, J. (1993). *The Celestine prophecy: An adventure*. New York: Warner Books.

Redfield, J. (1996). *The tenth insight: Holding the vision*. New York: Warner Books.

Remen, E. N. (1996). *Kitchen table wisdom: Stories that heal*. New York: Riverhead Books.

Rogers, M. E. (1964). *Reveille in nursing*. Philadelphia, PA: F. A. Davis.

Rogers, M. E. (1970). *An introduction to the theoretical basis of nursing*. Philadelphia, PA: F. A. Davis, Co.

Rogers, M. E. (1992). Nursing science and the space age. *Nursing Science Quarterly, 5*, 27–34.

Sabo, B. M. (2006). *Compassion fatigue and nursing work: Can we accurately capture the consequences of caring work? International Journal of Nursing Practice, 12*, 136–142.

Sack, K. (2010, February 10). Nurse to stand trial for reporting doctor. *The New York Times*. Retrieved from http://www.nytimes.com/2010/02/07/us/07nurses.html?pagewanted

Schantz, M. L. (2007). Compassion: A concept analysis. *Nursing Forum, 42*(2), 48–55.

Schaufeli, W. B., Leiter, M. P., & Maslach, C. (2009). Burnout: 35 years of research and practice. *Career Development International, 14*(3), 204–220.

Schluter, J., Winch, S., Holzhauser, K., & Henderson, A. (2008). Nurses' moral sensitivity and hospital ethical climate: A literature review. *Nursing Ethics, 15*, 304–321.

Schmalenberg, C., & Kramer, M. (2008). Clinical units with the healthiest work environments. *Critical Care Nurse, 28*(3), 65–77.

Schneiderman, L. J., Jecker, N. S., & Jonsen, A. R. (1990). Medical futility: Its meaning and ethical implications. *Annals of Internal Medicine, 112*(12), 949–954.

Schuster, M. A. et al. (2001). A national survey of stress reactions after the September 11, 2001 terrorist attacks. *New England Journal of Medicine, 345*(20), 1507–1512.

Shulman, L. S. (2009). [Foreword]. In P. Benner, M. Sutphen, V. Leonard, & L. Day (Eds.), *Educating nurses: A call for radical transformation*. Kindle version (Location 112–193). San Francisco: Jossey-Bass/Carnegie Foundation for the Advancement of Teaching. Kindle Edition. Retrieved from www.amazon.com

Scott, D. E. (2008). Nursing that works: Happiness at work. *New Jersey Nurse, 38*(6), 3, 9.

Smith, M. C. (1999). Caring and the science of unitary human beings. *Advances in Nursing Science, 21,* 14–28.

Smith, M. C. (2010). Marlaine Smith's theory of unitary caring. In M. E. Parker, & M. C. Smith (Ed.), *Nursing theories and nursing practice* (3rd ed., pp. 495–504). Philadelphia, PA: F A Davis.

Souba, W. W. (2002). Academic medicine and the search for meaning and purpose. *Academic Medicine, 77,* 139–144.

Stamm, B. H. (2002). Measuring compassion satisfaction as well as fatigue: Developmental history of the compassion fatigue and satisfaction test. In C. R. Figley (Ed.), *Treating compassion fatigue* (pp. 107–119). New York: Brunner Mazel.

Stamm, B. H. (2009). *Research Information on the ProQOL.* Retrieved from http:// www.compassionfatigue.org

Stamm, B. H. (2010). *The ProQOL (Professional Quality of Life Scale: Compassion Satisfaction and Compassion Fatigue).* Pocatello, ID: ProQOL.org. Retrieved from www.proqol.org.

Styles, M. M. (1992). Nightingale: The enduring symbol. In *F. Nightingale's Notes on nursing: What it is and is not. Commemorative Ed.* (pp. 72–75). Philadelphia, PA: J. B. Lippincott.

Thomas, S. P., & Burk, R. (2009). Junior nursing students' experiences of vertical violence during clinical rotations. *Nursing Outlook, 57*(4), 226–231.

Thoreau, H. D. (1854/1995). *Walden, or, life in the woods.* Mineola, NY: Dover.

Todaro-Franceschi, V. (1998). *The enigma of energy: A philosophical inquiry.* Doctoral dissertation, New York University (UMI No. 9819881).

Todaro-Franceschi, V. (1999). *The enigma of energy: Where science and religion converge.* New York: Crossroad Publishers.

Todaro-Franceschi, V. (2001). Energy: A bridging concept for nursing science. *Nursing Science Quarterly, 14,* 132–140.

Todaro-Franceschi, V. (2003). Letter to the editor. *Nursing Science Quarterly, 16,* 184–185.

Todaro-Franceschi, V. (2006). Synchronicity related to dead loved ones: A natural healing modality. *Spirituality and Health International, 7,* 151–161.

Todaro-Franceschi, V. (2007). Imagining nursing practice in the year 2050: Looking through a Rogerian looking glass. *Nursing Science Quarterly, 20,* 229–231.

Todaro-Franceschi, V. (2008a). Preventing compassion fatigue and reaffirming purpose in nursing. *Proceedings on the 3rd European Federation of Critical Care Nursing Congress and 27th Aniarti Conference, Influencing Critical Care Nursing in Europe,* Florence, Italy (Oct). Accessed at: http://www.aniarti.it/efccna2008/atti/10/mattino/sala2/pdf/5-todaro.pdf

Todaro-Franceschi, V. (2008b). Clarifying the enigma of energy, philosophically speaking. *Nursing Science Quarterly, 21,* 285–290.

Todaro-Franceschi, V. (2010). *Choices [A digital story].* Washington, DC: Author.

Todaro-Franceschi, V. (2011a). *Vestiges [A digital story].* Jackson, NJ: Author.

Todaro-Franceschi, V. (2011b). Changing the face of death: A pedagogic intervention. *Journal of Professional Nursing, 27*(5), 315–319.

Todaro-Franceschi, V. (2011c). Re-patterning health professional death education: A matter of social justice for all. *The Forum: The Quarterly Publication of the Association for Death Education and Counseling, 37*(3), 26–27.

Todaro-Franceschi, V. (2011d). *Remembering.* A digital story. Retrieved from http://www.youtube.com/watch?v=SB2EATOU0wo&context=C320c904 ADOEgsToPDskK9oh_kCfN3JWP6bHkRZcpi

Todaro-Franceschi, V. (2012). *A dying man and a chair. [A digital story].* Jackson, NJ: Author.

Tolle, E. (2005). *A new earth: Awakening to your life's purpose.* New York: A Plume Book.

Trinkoff, A. M., & Storr, C. L. (1998). Substance use among nurses: Differences between specialties. *American Journal of Public Health, 88*(4), 581–585.

Updegraff, J. A., Silver, R. C., & Holman, E. A. (2008). Searching for and finding meaning in collective trauma: Results from a national longitudinal study of the 9/11 terrorist attacks. *Journal of Personality and Social Psychology, 95*(3), 709–722.

Vachon, M. L. (1993). Emotional problems in palliative medicine: Patient, family, and professional. In D. Doyle, G. Hanks, & N. McDonald (Eds.), *Oxford textbook of palliative medicine* (pp. 577–605). New York: Oxford University Press.

Valent, P. (2002). Diagnosis and treatment of helper stresses, traumas and illnesses. In C. R. Figley (Ed.), *Treating compassion fatigue* (pp. 17–37). New York: Brunner-Routledge.

Valian, V. (2006). Women at the top in science-and elsewhere. In S. Ceci, & W. Williams (Eds.), *Why aren't more women in science?* (pp. 27–37). Washington, DC: American Psychological Association Press.

Vieten, C., Amorok, T., & Schlitz, M. M. (2006). I to we: The role of consciousness transformation in compassion and altruism. *Zygon, 41*(4), 915–931.

Volavkova, H. (Ed.). (1993). *I never saw another butterfly . . . .* New York: Schocken Books.

Watson, J. (1985). *Human science and human care.* Norwalk, CT: Appleton-Century-Crofts.

Watson, J. (1999). *Post modern nursing and beyond.* Edinburgh: Churchill.

Watson, J. (2008a). Nursing: *The philosophy and science of caring (Rev. ed.).* Boulder: University Press of Colorado.

Watson, J. (2008b). Caring science: Belonging before being as ethical cosmology. *Nursing Science Quarterly, 18,* 304–305.

Watson, J., & Woodward, T. K. (2010). Jean Watson's theory of human caring. In M. E. Parker, & M. C. Smith (Ed.), *Nursing theories and nursing practice* (3rd ed., pp. 351–369). Philadelphia, PA: F. A. Davis.

Weber, M. (1958). *Max Weber: Essays in sociology,* H. H. Gerth, & C. W. Mills (Eds. & Trans.). New York: Oxford University Press.

Weber, R. (1986). *Dialogues with scientists and sages: The search for unity.* New York: Routledge & Kegan Paul.

Webster, G., & Bayliss, F. (2000). *Moral residue.* In S. Rubin, & L. Zoloth (Eds.), *Margin of error: The ethics of mistakes in the practice of medicine.* Hagerstown, MD: University Publishing Group, Inc.

Wilkins, K., & Shields, M. (2008). Correlates of medication error in hospitals. *Health Reports, 19*(2), 7–18.

Wolf, G., Triolo, P., Reid-Ponte, P., Drenkard, K., & Moran, J. (2011). The next generation. In K. Drenkard, G. Wolf, & S. H. Morgan (Eds.), *Magnet: The next generation-nurses making the difference.* (pp. 23–30). Silver Spring, MD: American Nurses Credentialing Center.

Woodward, V. M. (1997). Professional caring: A contradiction in terms? *Journal of Advanced Nursing, 26,* 999–1004.

Woolf, V. (1922, February 17). *Diary.* Accessed at: http://www.readprint.com/author-91/Virginia-Woolf-books

Yarling, R. R., & McElmurry, B. J. (1986). The moral foundation of nursing. *Advances in Nursing Science, 8*(2), 63–73.

Yehuda, R. (2002a). Post-traumatic stress disorder. *New England Journal of Medicine, 346*(2), 108–114.

Yehuda, R. (Ed.). (2002b). *Treating trauma: Survivors with PTSD.* Washington, DC: American Psychiatric Publishing.

Zhang, B., Wright, A. A., Huskamp, H. A., Nilsson, M. E., Maciejewski, M. L., Earle, C. C., Block, S. D., Maciejewski, P. K., & Prigerson, H. G. (2009). Health care costs in the last week of life: Associations with end of life conversations. *Archives of Internal Medicine, 169*(5), 480–488.

INDEX